Second Edition

Patient Education

A Practical Approach

Kate Lorig
and Associates

SAGE Publications
International Educational and Professional Publisher
Thousand Oaks London New Delhi

For information address:

 SAGE Publications, Inc.
2455 Teller Road
Thousand Oaks, California 91320
E-mail: order@sagepub.com

SAGE Publications Ltd.
6 Bonhill Street
London EC2A 4PU
United Kingdom

SAGE Publications India Pvt. Ltd.
M-32 Market
Greater Kailash I
New Delhi 110 048 India

Printed in the United States of America

Library of Congress Cataloging-in-Publication Data

Lorig, Kate.
    Patient education: A practical approach / Kate Lorig.—2nd ed.
        p.   cm.
    Includes bibliographical references and index.
    ISBN 0-7619-0073-X (cloth: alk. paper).—ISBN 0-7619-0074-8 (pbk.: alk. paper)
        1. Patient education. I. Title.
    R727.4.L67 1995
    615.5é07—dc20   95-36414

This book is printed on acid-free paper.

96 97 98 99 10 9 8 7 6 5 4 3 2

Sage Production Editor: Diane S. Foster
Sage Typesetter: Andrea D. Swanson

Contents

Preface   ix

Acknowledgments   xi

Introduction   xiii
  Some Words and Definitions   xiii
  How to Use This Book   xv
  Problem List   xvi

1. **How Do I Know What Patients Want
   and Need? Needs Assessment**   1

    Kate Lorig

  Interested-Party Analysis   2
  Checklist Needs Assessment   4
  Salient Belief Assessment   5
  Matrix Assessment   8
  Focus Groups   10
  Structured/Semistructured Interviews   11
  Balanced Incomplete Block Design   12
  Epi Info—A Tool for Data Analysis   17

2. Do I Know Where To Go, and Will I Know When I Get There? Evaluation   19

Kate Lorig

Some Evaluation Words	20
Asking the Right Questions	25
Methods: How Do I Find Out What I Want to Find Out?	26
Finding and Choosing the Right Questions	30
Tips on Data Collection	35
Study Design	42
Appendix 2A. Patient Education Evaluation Scales	46
Visual Analogue Scales	47
Health Assessment Questionnaire	49
The Center for Epidemiologic Studies Depression Scale (CES-D)	58
Self-Reported Medication-Taking Scale	61
Group Health Association of America Consumer Satisfaction Survey	62

3. How Do I Get From a Needs Assessment to a Program? Program Planning and Implementation   67

Kate Lorig

Setting Priorities: Choosing What to Teach in the Time Allotted	68
Refining Your Content	71
Setting Objectives	71
Process	75
Who Will Teach the Program?	85
Knowing What to Teach and When to Teach	86
Knowing How to Teach	86
One-on-One Education	87
Group Education	88
Special Problems With Groups	89

Putting It All Together   90
Documenting What You Teach   95
Appendix 3A. Questions in Patient Education   97
Appendix 3B. Protocol for a Session of the
    Arthritis Self-Help Course   100

4. Selecting, Preparing, and Using Materials   117

    Cecilia Doak, Leonard Doak, and Kate Lorig

✱ Does the Material Contain the Information
    the Patient Wants?   118
✱ Does the Material Contain the Information
    the Patient Needs?   120
✱ Can the Patient Understand the Material
    as Presented?   121
Summary   129

5. How Do I Get People to Come?   131

    Virginia M. González and Kate Lorig

Marketing to Health Professionals   132
Marketing to the Public   136
Using Community Resources   146

6. Working Cross-Culturally   151

    Virginia M. González and Kate Lorig

Understanding Cultural Diversity   152
Where to Start   154
How Do I Create a Culturally Appropriate
    Program?   158
Strategies for Adapting Program Content
    and Process   160
Translation—More Than Meets the Eye   166
Conclusion   170

7. **Helping People Who Are Hard to Help**   **173**

    Kate Lorig

    Strong, Silent Types   174
    Talkers   176
    Antagonistic or Belligerent Participants   178
    "Yes, Buts"   179
    Attention Seekers   180
    Special Problem People   181

8. **The Special Problem of Compliance: How Do
    I Get People to Do What Is Good for Them?**   **183**

    Kate Lorig

9. **What We Know About What Works:
    One Rationale, Two Models, Three Theories**   **195**

    Jean Goeppinger and Kate Lorig

    Rationale: The Compression of Morbidity   197
    Three Theories: Self-Efficacy, Stress and
        Coping, and Learned Helplessness   198
    Two Models: PRECEDE and the Health
        Belief Model   216
    Conclusion   224

10. **Joint Commission on Accreditation of
     Healthcare Organizations (JCAHO):
     Patient and Family Education Regulations**   **227**

    Mary M. Hobbs

    Glossary   235

    Index   239

    About the Author   245

    About the Contributing Coauthors   247

Preface

This book is designed to solve problems, give practical advice, and build new skills. It is for health professionals who are not skilled in patient education but need to know where to start and how to proceed. It may also be useful to students who are just beginning to learn the tricks of the trade. If used as a text, it will take you step by step through the process of conceptualizing, designing, implementing, and evaluating patient education programs. It will also help you with JCAHO accreditation.

Over the past several years, I have been asked to give many patient education skills-building workshops. Some of these have been sponsored by the Veterans Administration and the American Hospital Association in the United States, others by the Arthritis Societies of New Zealand and Canada, the Arthritis Foundations of various states in Australia, and the Department of Rehabilitation at the University of Gothenberg in Sweden. Others have been sponsored by the Health Education Society in British Columbia and the Society for Public Health Education in Seattle, Washington. I have also been fortunate to consult with many fine colleagues in the Kaiser Permanente health care system.

During this same time, I have been running a Patient Education Research Center at Stanford University. This center has involved hundreds of community-based courses for thousands of people with arthritis and other chronic diseases, including heart disease, lung diseases, stroke, and AIDS. Our research has shown that patient education can change behaviors, improve health status, and save health care costs.

This book is a result of all the above activities. It is a collection of the bits and pieces designed for the workshops and reflects our experiences here at Stanford and the real-life experiences of the workshop participants. By including a large section on health education theory, I hope to help practitioners use theory in everyday practice. In short, this is a "how-to" guide to patient education that has grown out of my work over the past decade. I have tried to make suggestions that will have immediate relevance to practice. At the same time, many readers will want more information. This can be found in the short bibliographies at the end of each chapter.

Acknowledgments

Books don't just happen. This book is no exception. Over the years, many people have been very helpful. Milton Chernin was the first to suggest that I might write a book. I regret I was too slow to allow him to see the finished product. Many people have helped me learn about patient education. These include Carol D'Onofrio, Wendy Cuneo, Larry Green, Rusty Rosenstock, Charles Watson, Judith Miller, Barbara Giloth, Sam Radelfinger, Helen Ross, Rosemary Pries, David Sobel, and Mary Hobbs. Over the years, Godfry Hochbaum has given more wisdom and support than he will ever know.

For the past 16 years, I have had three Stanford mentors and colleagues who have supported my work, tried to keep me on track, and at the same time allowed me to explore uncharted territory. My very special thanks to Halsted Holman, James Fries, and Albert Bandura.

Added to these professionals are the hundreds of people who have attended patient education workshops I have given in the United States, Canada, Australia, New Zealand, South Africa, Singapore, and Sweden. You have asked important questions and have served as my guides for moving patient education from the ivory tower of academe to the clinical setting. In addition you have given me many ideas based on your practice.

Finally, there is a group of friends and colleagues who have written, typed, proofread, edited, critiqued, and in many other ways made this book more readable. My deepest appreciation to Diana Laurent, Virginia González, Jean Goeppinger, Cecilia and Leonard Doak, Larissa Ortiz, Bruce Campbell, Edith Superio, Jenny Davidson, Ian Fraser, and last but not least, Dr. Shapiro.

Introduction

¤ SOME WORDS AND DEFINITIONS

Throughout this book, I talk about "patient" education. The reason for using the word *patient* is that this is not a book about health promotion or disease prevention, although much from the book could be applied to such programs. Rather, it is about "patients"—people who have a defined health problem, be it high blood pressure, cancer, diabetes, or AIDS. Usually, when someone is receiving medical care for a condition, we call him or her a patient. This is especially true in hospitals and clinics. However, this same person with his or her illness is often found getting on with life in the community. In this case, he or she becomes a person with diabetes, high blood pressure, AIDS, or whatever. Somehow, saying "education for people with _____" is rather awkward. Thus, for literary purposes and to save trees, I will talk about patient education.

Patient education is any set of planned, educational activities designed to improve patients' health behaviors and/or health status. Notice, there is nothing in this definition about improving knowledge. Activities aimed at improving knowledge are patient teaching. Changes in knowledge may be necessary before we can change behaviors or health status. However, just because someone has correct knowledge does not mean he or she will change. If all we needed was knowledge, we would have no smokers, overweight people, or people eating high-cholesterol foods. Patient education is much more than knowledge change.

The purpose of patient education is to maintain or improve health, or, in some cases, to slow deterioration. The means by which this occurs are changes in behaviors and/or mental attitudes. Increased compliance with medication taking, decreased pain, shorter hospital stays, and decreased depression are all reasonable goals for patient education programs.

In recent years, patient education has become even more complex because it is no longer enough for patients to learn and practice specific skills. Rather, patients must self-manage their own diseases. Self-management differs in that it assists patients in gaining skills and, more important, in gaining the confidence to apply these skills on a day-to-day basis. It also assists the patient with changing roles and changing emotions. The three most distinguishing features of the self-management model are (a) dealing with the consequences of disease—illness, not just the physiological disease; (b) being concerned with problem solving, decision making, and patient confidence, rather than prescription and adherence; and (c) placing patients and health professionals in partnership relationships. Health professionals are primarily responsible for the medical management of the disease, and the patient is primarily responsible for the day-to-day management of the illness. The key to full partnership is continual patient/health professional communication.

Now that we have defined *patient* and *patient education,* there is one term left—*planned educational activities.* Patient education does not just happen; it is planned. This book is about the planning of patient education activities.

¤ HOW TO USE THIS BOOK

Being a patient educator is a little like being a Jack or Jill of all trades. Often you are called upon to design something such as a program or a one-on-one intervention. Other times you are asked to fix something—to answer questions such as "Why don't people come to my program?" or "Why don't the patients do what I tell them to do?" Still other times, you are asked to evaluate patient education. Another role is that of supplying resources: answering questions such as "Where do I get information on Parkinson's disease?" or "Where can I get a slide projector?" Finally, you may be asked to help prepare your facility for accreditation. Sometimes you are expected to put all of these roles together and create, implement, and evaluate an entire program. This book is designed to assist you with all these roles. Each chapter is aimed at a specific function or problem. Unlike most books, this one does not need to be read from beginning to end. Instead, there are several ways you can get started:

- As with any other book, start with the table of contents and read what you want.
- Start with the following problem list. The chapter numbers after the problem show where you will find answers.
- As you read, you will be directed to other parts of the book for more information on related subjects.

All of this is to say that there are many roads to a good patient education program. Try whichever one is best for you.

¤ PROBLEM LIST

1. Doctors will not:
   - Participate: Chapter 5
   - Refer: Chapter 5
   - Do what I want them to do: Chapter 5
2. Patients are not motivated: Chapters 1, 3, 5, 8, 9
3. Patients will not come: Chapter 5
4. We give the education and people don't change: Chapters 3, 7, 8, 9
5. Patients will not comply: Chapter 8
6. I do not have time: Chapter 3
7. How do we educate _____ (fill in any racial or ethnic group)? Chapters 4, 6
8. All that theory stuff does not make any sense in my "real" world: Chapter 9
9. I do not know if what I do makes a difference: Chapter 2
10. I do not have the resources to do patient education: Chapter 5
11. I do not know what to teach: Chapters 1, 3
12. How do I deal with talkative, quiet, belligerent, etc., patients? Chapter 7
13. How do I assess learner readiness and skill level? Chapters 1, 4
14. How do I deal with groups when people come with different knowledge, skills, and interests? Chapters 1, 3
15. How can I get over administrative barriers? Chapters 1, 2, 5
16. There is not enough space for classes: Chapter 5
17. How do I work with patients from other cultures? Chapter 6
18. How do I prepare written materials? Chapter 4
19. How do I choose materials? Chapter 4
20. The marketing department wants to change my program to meet marketing needs: Chapter 5
21. How do we prepare to meet the JCAHO patient and family education requirements? Chapter 10

How Do I Know What Patients Want and Need?
Needs Assessment

Kate Lorig

Programs that educate patients do not just happen. Rather, they are shaped by the beliefs and skills of those offering the education. All programs start with someone who believes that patients should know or do something. The program is then formed to ensure that this happens. The initial belief is the foundation of the program. The strength of the foundation, and thus of the whole program, is determined by how well the program fits the needs of those it will serve. Unfortunately, health professionals alone are usually not able to understand patient needs fully, and many programs fall short. Solid patient education programs, however, are built on carefully executed *needs assessments*.

Before discussing how to conduct needs assessments, here is a tip on how to get others in your organization to accept the idea of doing them. Often someone will come to you with an idea. You should make a pamphlet, put up a poster, or put together a class. The originator of the idea also knows exactly what should be written or taught. For whatever reason, you do not think this is a good idea. Rather than arguing, you can say, "It is our policy always to conduct a needs assessment, or to test new materials. Let us do this with your idea and see what happens." This approach changes your role from opponent to assistant. The following are several methods of conducting needs assessments.

¤ INTERESTED-PARTY ANALYSIS

One of the most common errors in planning any new program is not considering the needs of all those involved. Although it is evident that client needs are important, we often forget the needs of the other interested parties. There are often many such persons, including the patient's family, health professionals, friends, neighbors, other service agencies, and even marketing departments. Once the general topic of a program has been determined (e.g., cancer, diabetes, AIDS, or caregiver support), it is important to make a list of all the interested parties.

The next step is to interview the key people to find out what they want from your program and how this program may affect other programs. For instance, the fund-raising branch of the organization may see the program as a source of new donors or of special interest to a new donor community. On the other hand, they may be concerned about advertising for your program at the same time that they are pursuing another large public campaign. Furthermore, the volunteer recruiter may be overwhelmed by the need to recruit and train an additional 40 volunteers or may be overjoyed because your program will serve as a new recruiting tool. The assessment may have shown a need to provide services to a special language or cultural group. However, agency administration may be concerned that this would necessitate the hiring of bilingual staff, which could affect the budget. The marketing department may see your program as a way of attracting new clients.

Other agencies in the community may also have an interest in your plans. A program to assist the adult children of aging parents may be offered by other organizations or health providers. Your agency may find itself in a turf battle that could lead to unfavorable publicity.

Finally, the needs of clients may be different from the needs of their families. Children undergoing chemotherapy may see teasing by peers as a major problem. Thus the agency could provide a teasing-inoculation program by showing parents how to help their children gain new skills and confidence to manage the teasing or by working with the children directly. However, such a program would completely ignore the needs of parents of children with cancer, who must deal with family stress and the fear of future prognosis. Because most health problems affect not only the individual but also the family and community, it is important to get input from everyone before deciding the program focus.

Table 1.1 shows a suggested interview or questionnaire format for an interested-party analysis. Remember, it is not etched in stone and is offered as a guide for you to change and use as you wish.

You may want to ask other questions during this same interview, such as the best format, place, or time for the program or how to fund the program. However, these questions are not necessary in the needs assessment stage and are sometimes best left until you know exactly where you are going.

TABLE 1.1 Suggested Interview/Questionnaire Format for an Interested-Party Analysis

1. Name: _____
2. Reason for interviewing: _____. (For example, is this person a patient, a family member, an agency administrator?)
3. We are considering starting a _____ program and would be interested in your opinions. Because you are a _____, your ideas are very important.
4. Considering your position, what do you think should be the objective of the program? (For clients and their families, this question can be rephrased to "When you think of _____, what do you think of?")
5. What advantages do you see in starting this program?
6. What are the disadvantages or other possible problems that you foresee?
7. How do you see yourself (your agency) participating in this program?
8. Do you have any other thoughts that you would like to share with us?

¤ CHECKLIST NEEDS ASSESSMENT

Probably one of the most common forms of needs assessment is a questionnaire checklist. All you do is list a number of topics and let potential participants check off topics of interest. There are many advantages to this method. Checklists are easy to administer and to tally, and clients seldom object to them. However, checklists should not be used as the sole means of getting information. The problem is that a checklist usually reflects what professionals are ready to teach, not necessarily the interests of the patients. For example, many checklists about cardiac problems include such things as exercise, diet, and medication but fail to mention the problems of living with uncertainty. Yet we know from studies that uncertainty is usually a major concern for those patients. Why is it forgotten? Because living with uncertainty is not the central focus of any one health profession and therefore sometimes falls through the cracks.

Many checklists do have an "other" space. But there are seldom enough similar "other" responses to make these an important program-planning consideration. Still, all is not lost. Checklists can be useful if carefully constructed. The topics to be included should come from both patients and professionals. Focus groups are sometimes useful in writing checklists (see the section on focus groups later in this chapter). Be sure not to change or misrepresent the patient-generated items—for example, by changing "living with uncertainty" to "living with frustration."

All in all, it is probably best not to rely solely on checklists. But if you do, be sure to follow the above guidelines.

¤ SALIENT BELIEF ASSESSMENT

From psychology, we learn that human beings can have only seven or so beliefs or opinions about any one subject. These have been called *salient beliefs* (Fishbein & Ajzen, 1975; Miller, 1956). If you can identify these beliefs, you can use this knowledge as a basis for your educational efforts. Assessing salient beliefs is an especially useful strategy for the busy health care provider in one-on-one situations. A simple way of soliciting these beliefs is to ask the patient, "When you think of _____, what do you think about?" The blank can be filled in with any behavior or disease (e.g., exercise or cancer). The answers that you get will give you good insight into that person's beliefs and concerns about that particular condition or behavior.

People with arthritis most often answer the above question with "pain, disability, and depression." Knowing this, the health educator can then build a group or individual teaching program around managing pain and preventing disability. If the patient's first response is "fear," then the teaching should be aimed at determining the reason for the fear and trying to overcome it.

If the health educator wishes to establish a group program, a number of people with a similar condition or problem can be asked, "What do you think of when you think about _____?" They are asked to write as many answers to the question as they wish. These answers are then rated, with the first answer getting 10 points, the second answer 9 points, and so on. The total score is then added for each response. The responses with the highest scores are the most important for that group. Table 1.2 provides an example of how to do this scoring.

One of the advantages of this technique is that it enables you to tailor the education to the perceptions and needs of the patients. For example, most traditional cardiac rehabilitation education does not directly address uncertainty, but instead focuses on exercise, medication, and diet, which are the major concerns of health professionals working with coronary disease. These topics are all very important, but may be better accepted by patients if taught in the context of being better able to live with uncertainty.

A third way of using a salient belief assessment is for public lectures. Often we are asked to come and talk to a group about one topic or another. Because this is a one-shot song and dance, we generally show a film or give a lecture. Instead, we might start the presentation by saying something like this:

> We could say lots of things about AIDS, such as what it is, who can get it, how you get it, how you prevent it, or what safe sex is. Before beginning, I want to know what you would like to know about AIDS. I will make a list, and then we will vote on how you would like me to use my time.

TABLE 1.2 Scoring a Salient Belief Assessment for the Question, "What Do You Think of When You Think of Menopause?"

| | *Responses by Individual* | | | | | |
	Mary	*Score*	*Jane*	*Score*	*Rebecca*	*Score*
First response	hot flashes	10	sagging body	10	fatigue	10
Second response	growing older	9	no birth control	9	hot flashes	9
Third response	no menstruation	8	dry vagina	8	getting old	8
Fourth response	loss sex appeal	7	fatigue	7	fatigue	7

| *Aggregate Responses* | |
Response	*Total Score*
Hot flashes	$10 + 9 = 19/3 = 6.3$
Growing older	$9 + 8 = 17/3 = 5.7$
No menstruation	$8/3 = 2.7$
Loss of sex appeal	$7/3 = 2.3$
Sagging body	$10/3 = 3.3$
No birth control	$9/3 = 3$
Dry vagina	$8/3 = 2.7$
Fatigue	$7 + 7 + 10 = 24/3 = 8.0$

Priority for Teaching	*Score*
1. Fatigue	8.0
2. Hot flashes	6.3
3. Growing old	5.7

NOTE: These data are fictional and do not necessarily represent what should be taught about menopause.

At this point, ask the audience what they would like you to address. Write down all the items without comment, and then read the list. Next, give everyone two or three votes, and go through the list, having the audience vote. Finally, address your talk to the top three or four items on the list.

This technique has several advantages. First, it involves the audience and lets them know that you are really interested in their input. Second, it allows you to address the issues of special interest to that group. One reason some speakers are afraid to

try this technique is that they think the audience will ask
something that they are not prepared to address. Of course this
can happen, in which case all you have to do is say that you
don't know anything about how monoclonal antibodies affect
AIDS and go on to the next topic. Most of the time, however,
the topics chosen by the audience will be well known to you.

¤ MATRIX ASSESSMENT

This technique is especially good with a small group of no
more than 15 to 20 people. It is a quick variation on nominal
group process or the Delphi process (McKillip, 1987). First, ask
everyone to write a list of what he or she would like to learn in
the class. Make clear that these lists are for reference only and
will not be turned in. By having people write their individual
needs first, you are assured that everyone can participate and
that less popular needs will not get lost.

Ask the first person to read his or her list. Put each item in
a column heading at the top of a large blank matrix, and put
the person's name as the first row heading at the side of the
matrix. Then put an X by each item in his or her row. Put the
name of the second person as the next row heading. Put an X
by all the items that he or she names for which there are
headings at the top. Then give each new item a new column,
and add X's in the appropriate columns (see Figure 1.1).
Continue this process for each person in the group. After
everyone has exhausted his or her list, ask if anyone wants to
add any X's anywhere on the matrix. Some of the ideas of later
people may appeal to the earlier people. Finally, add all the X's
in each column. The topics with the most X's are the topics of

	How to Overcome Disabilities	Choosing a Doctor	Speech Problems	Controlling High Blood Pressure	Nutrition	Smoking	Stress Management	How to Choose a Nursing Home
John	X	X	X	X				
Maria		X	X	X	X		X	
Debbie	X				X	X		
Stan	X	X		X				
Pat	X						X	
Moses	X			X		X		
Joan		X			X			
Sasha	X	X		X				
Barbara	X				X			X
Jim	X	X					X	
Total	7	7	2	5	4	2	3	1

Figure 1.1. Matrix Assessment Chart for a Class for Stroke Patients

most interest and should be emphasized. This process also allows all the participants to see how their interests fit with the others in the group. If there is one person with very different interests, he or she may decide that this is not the appropriate group or may decide to stay without expectations of having his or her specific interests met.

¤ FOCUS GROUPS

A fifth way of conducting needs assessments is to get to-gether a small number of potential clients. Any number from 8 to 12 is ideal (Breitrose, 1988). It is important that the participants in the focus groups be like the people you are trying to reach. Focus groups usually work best if participants are similar. Thus, if you are trying to reach a very mixed audience, you might have several focus groups: one for the elderly women, another for the middle-aged men, and yet another for members of an ethnic minority community. Start by asking participants about their opinions. The secret is to be as nondirective as possible. For example, you might start by conducting a matrix assessment and then ask the focus group participants to discuss in more detail exactly what they would like to learn.

Another way to use a focus group is following a question-naire. For example, you learn that stroke patients would like an exercise videotape for home use. A focus group could then be used to determine the types of exercise desired, the length of the tape, willingness to buy the tape, and so on.

Brainstorming can also be used to start a focus group. (For more information, see the section on this topic in Chapter 3.)

Some notes of caution about focus groups: First, you may get only the opinions of the dominant group members. Other group members may not offer their opinions for fear of rejec-tion. For this reason, the person leading the focus group must have excellent group skills.

It is important that the group leader be an impartial person without ideas on—or, better yet, without knowledge of—the topic being discussed. If group leaders have strong opinions about the topic, it is very easy for them to lead the group, consciously or unconsciously, toward these ideas.

Focus group data are hard to interpret. As a leader or observer, you tend to hear what you want to hear. This is why it is important to have an impartial note taker to transcribe everything that takes place. Better yet, type and transcribe the focus group discussion. If you do this, have each person give his or her name every time he or she speaks. This makes the tape easier to transcribe. In reading the transcripts, see how many different people voice agreement or disagreement with an idea, not how often the idea is discussed. Often a dominant person will take up a good deal of time discussing an idea about which there is no agreement.

One way to use focus group data is to incorporate them into a further assessment using an incomplete block design evaluation (see the section on balanced incomplete block designs later in this chapter).

¤ STRUCTURED/SEMISTRUCTURED INTERVIEWS

Another way of conducting needs assessments is through an interview. For this, you make an interview format similar to that shown in Table 1.3. A group of people like those you are trying to reach are all interviewed using the same format. These interviews can be done in person or by phone. Our experience suggests that phone interviews are usually just as effective as face-to-face interviews and much more efficient. In addition, the phone allows you to interview people you could not reach in person. Of course, if the people you wish to reach do not have phones, face-to-face interviews are necessary. Public opinion polls are good examples of the use of structured interviews.

Structured interviews are good in that, like checklists, they are easy to administer and tally. In addition, you have the opportunity to clarify anything you do not understand. The disadvantage, as with checklists, is that you will never discover

TABLE 1.3 Sample Semistructured Interview

---

1. When you think of diabetes, what do you think of? (Note: This is a salient belief question.)
2. What are your greatest problems in living with diabetes?
3. Would you attend a 6-week class on diabetes?
   If yes:
      3a. Where should it be held?
      3b. What times are best for you?
      3c. What topics would you like covered?
   If no:
      3d. How would you like to learn about diabetes?
4. What would you like to know about diabetes?
5. What else about your diabetes would you like to tell us?

---

concerns that the interview does not cover. One way to get around this is by adding some open-ended or semistructured questions to your structured interview. If you do this, the open-ended questions should come before the structured questions. This helps prevent getting the answers the participants think you want to hear.

¤ BALANCED INCOMPLETE BLOCK DESIGN[1]

Many of the needs assessment techniques we have discussed—salient belief assessments, focus groups, and semistructured interviews—result in data that are somewhat hard to interpret. The use of an incomplete block design analysis helps solve this problem. Although this second-level assessment makes the process more complex, it results in data that are prioritized so that you know not only the priority but also the strength of the priority. For important patient education projects, the resulting information is well worth the effort.

TABLE 1.4 Sample List for Block Design: Elements in Chronic Disease Self-Management Course

1. Exercise	Starting an exercise program; learning how to monitor exercise
2. Medication	Proper use of medications
3. Symptom Management	Using the mind for symptom management (e.g., relaxation, visualization)
4. Communicating With Doctors	Improving interactions with doctors and other health professionals
5. Problem Solving	Learning to identify problems and to use techniques such as brainstorming to solve problems
6. Self-Confidence	Gaining self-confidence about being able to manage symptoms
7. Sharing	Sharing experiences with other students and learning from them

The balanced incomplete block design technique offers a very efficient means to rank items in a list through a series of forced comparisons. It produces a weighted ranking that shows the relative importance of each item in the list. It allows comparison of content and process items.

In the technique, all items are compared to one another using several sets of items (typically three or four per set). Subjects are asked to order each set from "most" to "least" (e.g., "most important" to "least important"). The rank order is obtained by summing the ranks assigned to each item.

The steps of doing a balanced incomplete block design study are as follows:

1. *List items.* List items to be ranked. This list is developed from the themes that emerged from your focus group or semistructured interviews. Typically, two or three people read the transcript of the focus group or interviews and then agree on themes. Table 1.4 lists seven elements in a patient education program.

TABLE 1.5 Some Balanced Incomplete Block Designs

Design A, for 7 Items	Design C, for 13 Items
1. Items 1, 2, 4	1. Items 1, 4, 5, 12
2. Items 2, 3, 5	2. Items 2, 5, 6, 13
3. Items 3, 4, 6	3. Items 3, 6, 7, 1
4. Items 4, 5, 7	4. Items 4, 7, 8, 2
5. Items 5, 6, 1	5. Items 5, 8, 9, 3
6. Items 6, 7, 2	6. Items 6, 9, 10, 4
7. Items 7, 1, 3	7. Items 7, 10, 11, 5
	8. Items 8, 11, 12, 6
Design B, for 9 Items	9. Items 9, 12, 13, 7
1. Items 1, 2, 3	10. Items 10, 13, 1, 8
2. Items 4, 5, 6	11. Items 11, 1, 2, 9
3. Items 7, 8, 9	12. Items 12, 2, 3, 10
4. Items 1, 4, 7	13. Items 13, 3, 4, 11
5. Items 2, 5, 8	
6. Items 3, 6, 9	
7. Items 1, 5, 9	
8. Items 2, 6, 7	
9. Items 3, 4, 8	
10. Items 1, 6, 8	
11. Items 2, 4, 9	
12. Items 3, 5, 7	

2. *Select design.* Count the number of items in your list and select the appropriate block design, using Table 1.5. Each design consists of a series of questions in which the respondent is asked to rank-order three or four items from the list in terms of their importance. In our sample list in Table 1.4, there are seven items, so we will use Design A. If the number of items in your list is not given in Table 1.5, you will have to construct your own block design. See Weller and Romney (1988).

3. *Create form.* Create a form, using the block design and your list of items. The form should contain instructions and a series of questions that group items according to the block design. See Figure 1.2 for our sample form. Our series of questions is con-

Chronic Disease Self-Management Assessment

NAME _____

DATE _____

We are interested in finding out how you rate the relative importance of various aspects of the proposed course. For the sets numbered 1 to 7 below, please mark each of the three items from most important (1) to least important (3).

As an example, consider ranking the colors blue, red, and green. If your favorite color among this group is red, you would place a "1" in the blank next to "Red" (see below). If your second favorite is green, you would place a "2" next to "Green" and a "3" next to "Blue."

___Blue	___Red	___Green

1.	___Exercise	___Medication	___Communicating with doctors
2.	___Medication	___Symptom management	___Problem solving
3.	___Symptom management	___Communicating with doctors	___Self-confidence
4.	___Communicating with doctors	___Problem solving	___Sharing
5.	___Problem solving	___Self-confidence	___Exercise
6.	___Self-confidence	___Sharing	___Medication
7.	___Sharing	___Exercise	___Symptom management

Figure 1.2. Sample Needs Assessment Form Using Block Design

structed from our item list and Design A. For example, the first question asks the respondent to rank-order Items 1, 2, and 4.

4. *Administer form.* This can be done either orally or in writing. We recommend the written form. For suggestions on the oral form, see Weller and Romney (1988).

TABLE 1.6 Ranking Study Tally Sheet

Category	1	2	3	Sum	N	Score
1. Exercise	111	11	1	10	6	1.6
2. Medication						
3. Symptom management						
4. Communication with doctors						
5. Problem solving						
6. Self-confidence						
7. Sharing						

5. *Tabulate results.* Tabulate results by summing ranks assigned to each item. To find the mean, divide the sum by the number of respondents. One method of tabulation is shown in Table 1.6.

One note of caution in doing needs assessments: If you already know what you are going to do and have no intention of changing, do not conduct a needs assessment. Nothing makes people angrier than being asked their opinions and then having those opinions ignored.

In conclusion, we have examined several ways of conducting needs assessments. There are also many other ways, including surveys, attitude-behavior-belief scales, and sampling. There is no one right or wrong way. Rather, you should use the method or methods that best fit your situation and will give you the information you need to know.

Patient education is not a science; there is no exact formula. It is an art, and thus it is up to you to mix and match methods to achieve the best program for your situation.

¤ EPI INFO—A TOOL FOR DATA ANALYSIS

The preparation and analysis of data can be made much easier by the use of a public-domain software product called Epi Info. This program was written at the Center for Disease Control in Atlanta, Georgia, and was originally intended for the use of public health officials investigating outbreaks of infectious disease. Despite its specialized beginnings, Epi Info is a versatile tool for the preparation of questionnaires of all kinds. Answers to questions can be entered on the computer and automatically added to a database. The resulting information can be analyzed with a variety of statistical tests and can be printed out in tabular or graphical form.

Epi Info includes its own word processor, but questions can be prepared on standard office word-processing programs and transferred to Epi Info. Questionnaire data can be exported to other spreadsheet, database, or statistical analysis programs (such as SPSS).

Perhaps the best thing about Epi Info is that the software program is inexpensive. The latest version (Epi Info 5) costs about $35 and can be ordered from USD Inc., 2156-D West Park Court, Stone Mountain, GA 30087, phone (404) 469-4098. One drawback is that Epi Info is currently available only for IBM-compatible computers.

¤ NOTE

1. Campbell, et al., Balanced incomplete block design: Description, case study, and implications for practice, *Health Education Quarterly,* 22(2), 201-210, copyright © 1995 by Sage Publications, Inc. Reprinted by permission.

¤ BIBLIOGRAPHY

Breitrose, P. (1988). *Focus groups—When and how to use them: A practical guide.* Palo Alto, CA: Stanford University, Health Promotion Resource Center.

Campbell, B. F., Sengupta, F., Santos, C., & Lorig, K. R. (1995). Balanced incomplete block design: Description, case study, and implications for practice. *Health Education Quarterly, 22*(2), 201-210.

Fishbein, M., & Ajzen, I. (1975). *Belief, attitude, intention and behavior.* Reading, MA: Addison-Wesley.

McKillip, J. (1987). *Need analysis: Tools for the human services and education.* Newbury Park, CA: Sage.

Miller, G. A. (1956). The magical number seven, plus or minus two: Some limits on our capacity for processing information. *Psychological Review, 631,* 81-87.

Morgan, D. L. (1988). *Focus groups as qualitative research.* Newbury Park, CA: Sage.

Weller, S., & Romney, A. (1988). *Systematic data collection.* Newbury Park, CA: Sage.

Do I Know Where to Go, and Will I Know When I Get There?
Evaluation

Kate Lorig

When you have completed the first step of developing a patient education program, needs assessment, your second step—though it may not be intuitively apparent—is evaluation. In planning a good program, you must consider evaluation early. It is an important step in clarifying program goals. All too often, evaluation is an afterthought, not an integral part of program planning. This chapter examines the questions to ask, types of evaluations, and evaluation design. By considering evaluation early, you can avoid problems and shape your program toward the outcomes you are trying to achieve. Let us look at some examples of evaluation as an afterthought:

- I wonder if our stop-smoking program was successful. We know that one year after the program we had a 30% quit rate. However, we do not have a control or comparison group (we just did not think about it soon enough). Therefore we do not know if 30% is good or bad. (In fact, this is an average or better one-year quit rate.)
- I sure would like to ask the mothers who came to our children's health fair what they found most useful. Unfortunately, I do not have any way of contacting them. In fact, I do not even know who came—just how many.
- I wonder if people who were referred to our weight loss program by doctors lost more weight than those who answered advertisements in the newspaper. However, I do not know how people learned about the program.
- People who took our diabetes course seem to be hospitalized less. I wish I had data to prove this. Our hospital administrator would be impressed by a cost-effective program.

Before discussing more about evaluations, let us discuss some of the basic vocabulary and concepts. Please do not skip this section. By being able to speak the same language and truly understand the concepts, you will not be thrown off base when someone challenges your evaluation as "subjective" and therefore not "valid."

¤ SOME EVALUATION WORDS

Many special terms are used to describe evaluations. These allow communication but are also sometimes used as a secret language or as a means of intimidation. The important thing to know is that there is no one right way to conduct evaluation. Rather, good evaluations are part art and part science. Even the very best evaluators are learning new things every day. The following are some common evaluation terms. Being familiar and comfortable with them should serve you well.

Process or Formative Evaluations

Process or *formative evaluations* ask questions about how your program is operating. In other words, you are evaluating the process. These evaluations can be very simple or quite complex. Process questions include: How many people attended? Where did people find out about the program? Were some classes better attended than others? What was the dropout rate? Were the people who dropped out like the people who stayed, or were they different? How did the people who participated differ from the general population? Process evaluations can also be used to find out if the program is being implemented according to a set protocol and if the teachers are liked by the participants.

Outcome or Summative Evaluations

Outcome or *summative evaluations* ask whether your program is doing what you wanted it to do. Most commonly, outcome evaluations ask questions about changes in behaviors, health status, or health care utilization. However, sometimes you may put on a program with the expressed purpose of improving patient satisfaction. If this is the *purpose* of your program, then satisfaction could be an outcome, although it is usually a measure of process. The key consideration is the *intended outcome* of your program and whether you are evaluating this.

Of course, if you are not clear about what you want a program to do, it is very hard to evaluate outcome.

Quantitative Evaluation

Quantitative evaluation collects data that are easily converted into numbers. It can be used for either a process or an outcome evaluation. Examples of quantitative evaluations are

- Asking participants to rate instructors on set scales
- Using instruments to measure depression, satisfaction, disability, etc.
- Using clinical data such as blood pressure or blood glucose
- Using chart or self-report data on utilization, such as the number of days in hospital or the number of emergency room visits

Quantitative evaluations are best used when you are very clear about the question that you want answered—that is, when you have a hypothesis. If you have a clear hypothesis, then almost anything can be quantified.

Qualitative Evaluation

Qualitative evaluation collects data that are not easily converted into numbers. (Even qualitative data can often be converted to numbers, but this takes thought and skill.) Qualitative data are almost always words. They are collected by means of semistructured interviews, focus groups, listening to the conversation of others, open-ended questions, or observation.

Qualitative evaluations are best when you are not at all clear about what is happening or when you do not know exactly what question to ask. These evaluations are often used to form a question or a hypothesis for a quantitative study.

To make things even more complicated, both quantitative and qualitative methods can be used in the same evaluation. For example, you might ask a series of questions about depression, health status, and behaviors, and then ask an open-ended question about what participants found most useful from an intervention.

Objective/Subjective

Objective and *subjective* are words that are often used to confuse or intimidate the beginning evaluator. In theory, *objective* refers to anything that can be verified by a standard test and outside observation. Such data as blood pressure, cholesterol levels, and number of visits to a doctor are considered objective. *Subjective* refers to any data that can be biased by or are the opinion of the reporter. Subjective data are considered not to be valid or "real" and are therefore suspect.

The problem is that the line between objective and subjective is not at all clear. Let us examine self-report of visits to physicians (considered by some to be subjective) as contrasted with chart audit (considered by some to be objective). It is true that an individual may over- or underreport the number of visits or may confuse a visit to a lab with a visit to a doctor. However, a chart audit may also have problems. The individual may see several doctors at different places, and not all the charts may be audited, leading to underreporting of visits. The person doing the chart audit may count as only one visit seeing a primary care physician and then being referred to a specialist on the same day. Thus chart audits are not always valid.

Other examples of objective data are blood pressure and cholesterol level. Many people have been declared hypertensive on the basis of blood pressure readings taken in a physician's office. In fact, the blood pressure may be high because of the anxiety surrounding a doctor visit. As for cholesterol level, laboratory data sent to five different labs have a good chance of getting several different cholesterol readings, some as much as 20 to 30 points apart.

The point is that seemingly objective data can be subject to bias. At the same time, subjective data can be valid. For example, pain and stress are always subjective. The important issue is not objective versus subjective, but rather whether the data are valid. Do not ever let anyone intimidate you by questioning the "objectivity" of your data. Be prepared to explain why you believe that the data are *valid*.

Valid

Valid is the key word when collecting any type of data. For data to be valid, they must meet two tests. First, you must get the same answers if you do the same test or ask the same questions twice within a short period of time. This is called *reliability*. However, something can be reliable without being true. For example, a clock is 15 minutes fast. Five people look at the clock and report the same time. The data are reliable, but they are not correct. For something to be valid, it must be both reliable and correct.

To determine the correctness or validity of data, we usually compare it with some "gold standard." For example, we have an individual self-report his or her disability and then have a physical therapist (PT) give the person a series of tests and report the disability. If the two reports are the same, then the self-reported data are usually considered valid because they are the same as the "gold standard" or the rating of the PT.

¤ ASKING THE RIGHT QUESTIONS

The most important part of any evaluation is asking the right questions. All evaluations start with the same two questions: (a) What do you want to know? and (b) Who cares? or, put more nicely, What difference does it make? It is important to spend a great deal of thought and time answering these two questions. As soon as you start to do an evaluation, you will think of a million things you would like to know. Then, just to complicate matters, all your colleagues will think of extra things that they would like to add to your evaluation. The result can soon become a 3-hour interview or a 50-page questionnaire. Stop! Decide three to five things that are the goals of your program and that you most want to know. Stick with these. There are several problems with collecting a lot of data. First, the longer the evaluation, the fewer the people who will complete it. Second, when you are finished, you are likely to be swimming in data, and you will not have enough time to analyze everything you have collected. In short, use the KIS principle—Keep It Simple.

The following patient education outcomes provide a general frame-work for deciding what you want to ask:

1. *Knowledge:* Did the participants learn what you wanted them to learn?
2. *Behaviors:* These are such things as exercise, medication compliance, communicating with physicians, and using an inhaler properly. Behavior measures answer the question "Are participants doing what you want them to do?"
3. *Attitudes/beliefs:* Have you changed patients' beliefs about the condition or their confidence (self-efficacy) in being able to do something about symptoms? Satisfaction with the health care system or with your intervention is also an attitude measure.

4. *Health status:* This is the real bottom line. Measures include blood pressure, disability, fatigue, shortness of breath, pain, role function, and blood glucose levels. A subset of health status measures would be psychological measures such as depression, anxiety, and health distress.

5. *Health care utilization:* Sample measures include number and type of outpatient visits, hospitalizations, days in hospital, use of medications, and emergency room use.

Once you have more or less decided the questions you want to ask, put them to the acid test. Ask yourself, "Who cares?" If you cannot give a clear, concise answer without beating around the bush, you probably do not have very good questions. By the way, when your colleagues come up with extra questions, you can use the same test. Ask them, "Who cares?" As a rule of thumb, if an interview or questionnaire takes more than 15 minutes to complete, it is probably too long. (Please note, this is not true if you are doing research as opposed to program evaluation.)

¤ METHODS: HOW DO I FIND OUT WHAT I WANT TO FIND OUT?

There are two basic evaluation methods: qualitative and quantitative. Some people might label these as subjective and objective evaluations. Do not get caught in this trap! If these words still confuse you, reread the discussion earlier in this chapter of the terms *objective* and *subjective.* There is nothing inherently subjective or objective about either method, nor is one method better than the other. Rather, the best evaluations use both methods. The question, not the bias of the evaluator, should be the basis for your choice of evaluation method.

Qualitative Evaluations

Qualitative methods are often used for answering "messy" questions. Sometimes we want to know why something happened: for example, why heart disease patients stopped smoking. One way of getting the answer is to make a list of all possible reasons and have the ex-smokers check off the answers. The problem here is that no one can make an all-inclusive list. You will get only the answers on your list, and you may miss the real reason that people stopped smoking. In this case, using qualitative methodology would probably be better. Just ask people why they stopped smoking. Then have three judges read all the answers and form a list of general categories. Compare the three lists of categories and form one list of categories. You should not have more than 10 to 12 categories in all. Now go back through all the answers and have each of the three judges fit every answer into a category. Finally, compare the category placements of the three judges. Hold a discussion until consensus is reached for any differences in opinion. If some responses do not fit a category, then form new categories. It is important that all responses fit a category. An "other" category does not count. Also, it is important that consensus is reached when there is a disagreement.

Now, you may think that this would be much easier if only one person did all the above steps. It is true that you would avoid disagreement, but you also might miss some of the most important material. For example, in a study of the problems of handicapped children in school, the children often mentioned problems with physical education courses. Two of the judges put these responses into a category of physical problems. However, the third judge, who had been a handicapped child, put these responses into the social problems category. She ultimately convinced the other judges to agree with her. As you can see, the solution to this problem is very different depending on whether you consider it a physical or social problem.

If the question is really important, you can take the themes generated by a qualitative study and use an incomplete block design questionnaire (see Chapter 1) to survey your population. This methodology combines the strengths of qualitative and quantitative methods to gather data about messy questions.

Generally, qualitative evaluations take more time than quantitative ones. However, they often result in perspectives that would have been lost if only quantitative data had been collected. Incomplete perspectives can lead to weak programs. For example, one evaluator doing a study of compliance asked cardiac patients how often they forgot to take their medications. She concluded that patients forgot 20% to 40% of the time, so she built a program based on memory aids. Another evaluator asked cardiac patients why they did not always take medications as directed, and found that medications were missed in social situations. They were also missed because of misinterpretation of symptoms. The patient felt better and therefore decided there was no need for the medication, felt worse and decided the medication was not helping, or suffered side effects and decided not to take the medication. Using these findings, the second evaluator based her program around rehearsal of medication taking in social situations and reinterpretation of symptoms. The second program is likely to gain greater compliance than the first.

In choosing between quantitative and qualitative evaluations, a good rule to follow is that if you are not sure what you need to know, use qualitative methods. Ask the people who know, usually the patients.

Very often when conducting evaluations, you ask questions of the wrong people or maybe not of enough categories of people. For example, sometimes you want to know why people drop out of classes or have very sporadic attendance. To find the answer, you often ask the instructors. Now, everyone has a legitimate reason for not coming to class—an aunt is visiting, they went on vacation, a child was sick. But unless people are very angry, they will never tell the instructor that they were bored, the room was uncomfortable, or their classmates had bad body odor. Thus, if you want to find out why people dropped out, call them and ask. A few carefully worded, tactful questions over the phone can get you a large amount of information. (By the way, the instructor should never be the one making these calls.)

One last point about asking qualitative questions. Experiment a little with wording. Remember that people do not generally like to be negative. Therefore, asking what participants did not like about the program will not elicit much information. Rather, ask what they would change in the program. Also, if you ask what people liked, the answer is often "everything." Again, this is not a very helpful answer. Instead, ask, "If you could attend only two or three parts of this program, what would you choose to attend?" or "If you could keep only three parts of the program, what would you keep?" This type of question forces participants to make a choice without being obnoxious. If you do not know how to ask a question, ask it three or four different ways and see which way yields the most useful (note, I did not say the most favorable) answers.

Quantitative Evaluations

Most evaluators favor quantitative evaluations, or those that collect numbers. These are generally easier to conduct, and somehow numbers seem more solid than opinions. In some cases this is true, and in others it is not. You would not ask someone to give you his or her opinion about his or her blood pressure reading; you would take his or her blood pressure. On the other hand, as we have already seen, valuable data are often lost in quantitative evaluations.

Usually, quantitative evaluations are conducted using a questionnaire, clinical data, or data that have already been collected for something else. Let us look at the latter first. Suppose that you want to conduct a hypertension program and want to know how many hypertensive patients there are in your institution. You might take the blood pressure of everyone who walks in the door for a week. This would give you some idea. An easier approach would be to go to the pharmacy and find out how many prescriptions are given out for hypertensive medications during the week. Both of these data collection methods have many flaws. Today, with increasingly sophisticated medical information systems, you might be able to get the computer to generate the number of patients seen for a specific problem. Be careful to find out the number of people, not the number of visits, as the latter measure may greatly exaggerate the number.

¤ FINDING AND CHOOSING
THE RIGHT QUESTIONS

In most quantitative evaluations, you need to ask one or more questions. The more questions you ask, the more burden you put on the responder (sometimes called *response burden*). In addition, the more questions you ask, the more data you have to clean, code, enter into a computer, and analyze. All this takes time. Therefore you are usually better off asking a few important, well-aimed questions than shotgunning and hoping you will hit something. It is very important to ask the "right" questions. In the following paragraphs, we examine how to locate and make decisions about which questions to ask. First, however, you should note Rule Number 1: *If at all possible, do not create your own questions!* Writing evaluation questions is an art and a science. It is usually done by people called psychometricians. Although this is a very useful skill, and can certainly be learned, it is probably more than the busy practitioner wants to tackle.

So if you are not going to write your own questions, how do you start?

First, you must be very clear about what you want to know. We discussed this earlier, but let us use some more examples. Say you want to know if someone has more "control" of his or her behavior or symptoms after an educational program. You must define *control*. The literature contains many control-related psychological constructs, such as coping, learned helplessness, locus of control, health locus of control, empowerment, and self-efficacy. Each has a different definition, and in fact each is different from the others. If you know only that you want to investigate "control," you are rather like the forest ranger who reports that she wants to count "animals"; when questioned, she reveals she is not interested in fish or insects, just four-legged animals, and upon more questioning, she realizes that what she really wants to know is the number of white-tailed deer living in a certain geographic area. You must be equally specific in deciding what you want to measure.

If you have only a general idea, go to the library and do some reading to help you narrow down your ideas. Talk with colleagues. The most important thing is to choose something you really want to know and define it clearly. This is called the *operational definition.*

Let us say you decide on self-efficacy but have no idea of how to measure it. You know from your previous work that self-efficacy is behavior-specific. Therefore, if you are evaluating an exercise program, you want questions about exercise self-efficacy.

To find an exercise self-efficacy *scale* (a group of related questions), conduct a search of Medline and Psychology Abstracts using the key words *exercise* and *self-efficacy*. If the resulting list is too long, narrow the search by adding the word *scale* or *instrument*. Look at the titles and abstracts to see if any of the articles describe an exercise self-efficacy scale. If not, see if there are one or two authors who have done several exercise self-efficacy studies. If so, call or write and ask what scales they use. Another thing you can do is to read some of the exercise self-efficacy studies. The instruments used for data collection are almost always described or referenced.

So you have done all of the above and now have not only one scale but four. How do you make a decision? Can you take the best questions from each?

Before answering these questions, we must again define some terms. A *question* is just that, one question. Sometimes one question will do: for example, "Check one: male ____ female ____." We would not, on the other hand, decide if someone could cope by asking the question "Can you cope?" For many outcomes, to get a really good answer we need a series of different but related questions. This series of questions is called a *scale* or an *instrument*. Sometimes, when we think we need only one question, using a scale may be more helpful. For example, in doing a study in a gay, bisexual, or transsexual community, we might ask:

1. What was your gender at birth? male ____ female ____
2. How do you identify yourself now? male ____ female ____
3. Have your external sex organs been surgically altered? yes ____ no ____

Having defined *question, scale,* and *instrument,* let us go to Rule Number 2: *Do not pick and choose questions or change questions.*

Scales must be used as a whole. The questions are like pieces of a jigsaw puzzle—they fit together. If a question or piece is missing, you get only part of the picture. Of course, as with everything else, there are exceptions.

Some scales have subscales. A coping scale may use different questions to measure cognitive coping, passive coping, and physical coping. When put together, these three subscales form a coping scale. If you are interested only in cognitive coping, you can use the cognitive coping subscale and forget the rest of the questions. Sometimes when you read about a scale, you will find it is made up of four subscales (sometimes termed *factors*). A factor is the same as a subscale. All the questions in a subscale or a factor relate to each other better than they do to another subscale. This is what one learns from a *factor analysis*.

As a general rule of thumb, do not change the wording of questions. Sometimes, however, you have to use common sense. For example, an American disability scale asks about the ability to turn off a faucet. This makes no sense in Australia, where a "faucet" is a "tap." In changing things you have to be *very* careful. This same scale, developed in the 1970s, asks about "dialing a telephone." Today, most people do not dial phones. However, changing the wording to "using a telephone" defeats the purpose of the original question, which is to determine finger and wrist function. The question might have to be changed to "turning a door knob" or "using a computer mouse."

Suppose you have found several scales and are not planning to change them. How do you choose which one to use?

First, let us assume that all the scales have been tested for reliability and validity (see the section "Some Evaluation Words," subsection "Valid," earlier in this chapter). If you cannot find information to confirm this, then the scale should be dropped from consideration.

Next, you should look at usability. Is the scale usable by the evaluator? If you are working with 20 to 30 subjects, the coding of a visual analogue scale, which requires measurement with a ruler, is fairly easy. However, if you have hundreds or thousands of subjects, visual analogue scaling will require extra time and resources. Can the data be entered into a computer by use of a scanner? Of course, if the answer is yes, you must consider the cost of a scanner, and then you must consider the ability of your population to fill out scanner sheets correctly. Does the scoring of the scale require complicated computer algorithms (decision charts), and if so, do you have someone who can create these? Is the coding straightforward or complicated? In general, the best advice is to keep it simple.

Probably more important is the user-friendliness of the instruments. Length is important. Generally, the more questions, the more missing data you will have. If you have too few questions, however, you may sacrifice validity or the ability to register change (sensitivity). Decisions should not be made on the basis of length alone. In one case, we tested two scales measuring the same thing. One scale had 6 questions and the other scale had 20 questions. Our population much preferred the 20-question scale because the responses (*once a week, twice a week,* etc.) were much more understandable than the responses on the shorter scale (*frequently, sometimes, seldom,* etc.).

Second, are the questions and the responses understandable to the people using the scale? You test this by trying out the scales on a few people and asking them if there are any problems.

Third, are the questions too personal, or do they anger people in some way? Are the questions relevant to the people answering them? Asking Hispanics in New York about their use of tortillas probably is not wise. However, asking about rice and beans, foods common in the Southwest, Mexican, Central American, and Caribbean Hispanic communities, may be more productive.

Finally, are the questions repetitive? Asking the same thing many different ways may increase your validity. At the same time, you may tire people or make them angry because they think you are trying to trick them.

Appendix 2A at the end of this chapter contains a variety of self-administered questionnaires that have been used for evaluating patient education programs.

¤ TIPS ON DATA COLLECTION

Data are essential for both needs assessment and evaluation. The results of these endeavors are only as good as your data. Therefore, if your data are not representative of the group or if they are incomplete, your results can be badly flawed. For example, if you want to know about patient satisfaction, and you hand out questionnaires in the waiting room, your sample is made up of only those who have sought care. You are missing all the people who may be so dissatisfied that they have gone elsewhere. It would be better to mail questionnaires or interview all patients (or a random sample of all patients) who were seen during a specified time period. Choosing a representative sample is not always easy, but it is necessary if you are to draw valid conclusions.

The biggest problem is often getting complete questionnaires. Sending out a questionnaire once is not enough. In our patient education studies, we mail our questionnaires with a friendly letter. Within 2 weeks, we usually get back about 50%. Then we send a postcard reminder, followed in about 10 days by a telephone call. Finally, 4 to 5 weeks after sending the initial questionnaire, we send a second questionnaire. This process usually results in an 80% to 90% return rate.

Getting back questionnaires, however, is only the halfway point in collecting good data. The other half involves getting complete data. Returned questionnaires are of little use if important parts of the questionnaire are not filled in correctly or are blank.

There are several ways to avoid this problem. First, formatting of the questionnaire is very important. The following are some suggestions:

1. Put questions on only one side of the page. If you must use both sides, be sure to cue your subjects to turn the page over.
2. When you have many lines of questions, shade every second or third line so that the people completing the questionnaire will not check off the wrong answer.
3. Do not try to shorten your questionnaire by using small type or compressing the questions. It is best to use size 12 or 14 type.
4. Put your questionnaires on colored paper (tan, yellow, pink) so that they are easy to find on a desk full of white papers. Use the same color for the whole evaluation.
5. Think of your coding before you print your questionnaire, and leave a space and lines for coding on the right side of the questionnaire. This is very important for computerized data entry. The entry persons should only have to read down the side of the page, not search out each answer. This process will also help you decide how to code answers and will help clarify what you really want to know and how to ask it. Good question-naire construction will save you many problems caused by missing data or data that are impossible to interpret.

Having said all this, no matter how well you construct your questionnaires, people will find a way to mess them up. This puts you in the position of having to recapture data.

If a whole page is missing, send the questionnaire back to the subject with a nice note asking them to complete the missing page. Be sure to keep a photocopy so you do not lose any data already in hand.

If you just have a few questions that need clarification, send the person a postcard asking him or her to call you during office hours. Keep the questionnaires near the phone in alphabetical order so they can be found easily. Much time can be saved by having people call you. Of course, you must be sure the phone is answered by someone trained to collect the missing data.

If after one week the person has not called, call him or her. Remember, many people work, so you might have to call in the early evening.

When you are collecting data from the same person more than once, you will need to find him or her a second time. To help with this, on your first questionnaire, ask for the name, address, and telephone number of someone who will always know where the subject is living. Then if the person gets ill, moves, or dies, you will have another point of contact to pursue when you are doing follow-up.

Some populations are harder to get data from than others. This is especially true for follow-up data. Here are a few ideas from practitioner friends:

1. For a community survey of parents of young children, a short questionnaire was placed on the back of tray mats at a fast food restaurant; the front side was left blank for artwork. Children were encouraged to draw a picture, and this was entered into a contest if the parents filled out the questionnaire on the back.

2. Women in jail were given a class on family planning and AIDS prevention. At the time of the class, they were asked for self-addressed envelopes to be used for follow-up questionnaires 6 months later. As an incentive for returning the questionnaire, each person was sent a state lottery ticket upon

return of the questionnaire. A surprising 55% of the population was found and responded.

3. A needs assessment was conducted with medical residents. As an incentive for filling out the questionnaire, the names of those returning the questionnaire were entered into a lottery for dinner at a fine restaurant.

Table 2.1 may help you avoid some common questionnaire pitfalls.

Finally you have all your data. Now what to do? Data analysis and statistics usually make the eyes of a patient educator glaze. Don't become catatonic. First there are some good, easy-to-use statistics books for beginners (Brown & Beck, 1994; Kanji, 1993). You might be surprised at what you can do yourself. Even without a statistics book, you can do averages and tallies. This may be enough. Thirty percent of the people stopped smoking for one year. The average class attendance was 4.2 out of 6 sessions. Participants lost an average of 5 pounds during the 10-week program.

Another useful tool for data analysis is Epi Info (see Chapter 1's final section for details). This inexpensive program for DOS-based computers is very user-friendly and comes with an excellent manual. The software is available for public access and thus can be freely shared.

Again, data analysis is a specialty for which you can get help. However, do not wait until the end of your project to talk with a statistician. The time to start talking is when you are beginning to think about evaluation. Statisticians are much more than number crunchers. If you get one interested in a project early, he or she can be a huge amount of help. Unfortunately, some statisticians do not speak English; they speak their own brand of professional jargon. If possible, avoid this type. By the way, you probably do not need a card-carrying statistician. Very

TABLE 2.1 What Can Go Wrong With Questionnaires—and Usually
              Does!

Problem	Possible Reason	Possible Solution
They don't return the form.	Takes too much effort to get it back.	Make it easier. Send a stamped envelope. If local, make the return point as central as possible or pick up the forms yourself. Send a short, friendly letter explaining the study and encouraging a quick response.
They didn't even do them!	People have a right not to participate.	Accept it or remind them with a postcard or phone call.
	May not be as interested in the topic as you are.	Jazz it up. Try to increase their motivation to participate.
	Didn't understand what you wanted.	Call to get responses to a few important questions. Keep things as clear as possible. People don't struggle to understand; they're more likely just to throw the questionnaire away. Provide a sample response. Really good pretests would have shown a problem here.
They didn't answer all the items.	Not time enough?	Don't rush them. Call them. Don't ask too many questions for the time allowed or for the effort it takes.
They left an answer blank.	Maybe some were uncomfortable about answering.	Try to eliminate unnecessary sensitive items. Try wording uncomfortable items carefully to minimize the reaction. May not be able to get at crucial stuff in the way; may need a relaxed, trusting interview.

continued

TABLE 2.1 Continued

Problem	Possible Reason	Possible Solution
	Maybe they didn't know what to answer, had not enough information, or had no opinion.	Ask questions your sample would be expected to know.
	Maybe you didn't give them the choice they wanted.	At least at pretest, and if possible at test, leave one "Other (specify) _____."
They cut off my secret identifying code.	People aren't as dumb as they used to be.	Be open with your identification. Ask them to sign; but it has to be voluntary. (You risk getting fewer returned.) Don't bank on knowing exactly who they are.
On follow-up questionnaires, you cannot find participants.	They moved away or are deceased.	On the first questionnaire, ask them to provide the name, address, and phone number of someone who will know their whereabouts in 1 to 5 years.
They marked too many answers.	Maybe the choices you gave were not mutually exclusive.	If the choices are of the same kind, try to combine them into a single answer that reflects both parts.
	Questions and answers may have been spaced too close together.	Sometimes you can figure out which is the most likely to be the answer.
	Some answers depend on different circumstances.	Be prepared to jettison items or whole forms for those problems.
	Your directions were not clear.	Be sure initial directions and even each page or item says how many to mark. But some people just won't follow directions anyway!

continued

TABLE 2.1 Continued

Problem	Possible Reason	Possible Solution
They added their own answer.	Maybe you forgot a whole category of answers.	Hope you can include that on the next go-around. It is better to get this on the pretest, but you can't always be so lucky. Try to fit their answer within existing categories.
Everybody marked the same answer.	You picked a skewed sample.	Unless it's contraindicated, look for balance in other groups.
	You didn't break the answers down far enough.	Remove the item for reworking, retesting, etc.
	You asked an obvious question.	Dumb!
	You just confirmed a major trend.	Publish your finding fast.
I don't think they answered honestly.	May be hostile to tests, the situation, you, etc.	Try to win their cooperation. Be ready to toss out obvious goof-ups.
	May have a sense of humor, be drunk, etc.	Ditto.
	May be guarding confidential material.	If it is vital to know, use double items to check reliability. Be prepared to lose items. Try to figure out why they'd want to lie and judge what to do accordingly. The bottom line is, trust people; they usually tell the truth.

continued

TABLE 2.1 Continued

Problem	Possible Reason	Possible Solution
Why didn't I think to ask just that one other question?	Even researchers aren't omniscient.	Try a new form. Set up a dummy conclusion as completely as you can *before* you give the test; using your imagination this way can often suggest an omitted item. Try a new group with it added. Better luck next time.
They took so long to return it.	You didn't put a return date on it.	Place the date by which you need it where it's sure to be seen. Send a reminder a week or so after the due date to remind those who have not yet returned them. (This is where it pays to know just who has returned and who has not returned questionnaires.)

SOURCE: Archer, Fleshman: *Community Health Nursing*, ©1985. Boston: Jones and Bartlett Publishers. Adapted with permission.
NOTE: Remember, always be nice; the participant is always right.

often someone with an advanced degree in one of the health sciences can help you.

¤ STUDY DESIGN

Like questionnaire design, study design is an art. There are several excellent books that will give you good ideas (see Green & Lewis, 1986; Windsor, Barabowski, Clark, & Cutter, 1994). The most important thing to remember is that quantitative evaluations need some type of comparison. Participants' condition after the program can be compared with their condition before the program. That is how we got the 30% quit rate for smokers. Sometimes participants are compared several times. For example, you get exercise rates 4 months before the program, when the program starts, 4 months later, 8 months later, and one year later. This is a time series design and has the advantage of letting you know two things. First, did your program cause the change in exercise rates, or was it caused just by time? You might find that 20% of the group started exercising in the 4 months before the program but that after the program, 70% of the group was exercising. This suggests that the program was responsible for getting 30% to 50% of the group to exercise. By continuing to collect data, you can find out how long program effects last. If at 8 months only 10% of the population is exercising, then the program's effect didn't last very long. However, if at one year 50% of the people are still exercising, you know that the program had a good long-term effect.

Usually, the strongest design is one that has a randomized comparison group. In this case, you would take all the people who were interested in a program and let half of them take the program while the other half were not allowed to take the program or were asked to wait for several months before taking the program. In this way, you can compare those taking the program with those not taking the program. When the two groups are randomly chosen, they are probably very similar. Therefore any effects that you find are likely to be caused by your intervention and not differences in the groups.

Most health education practitioners are reluctant to use a randomized design because they are afraid that those told that they cannot take the program will be angry. In reality, we have found that if people understand what you are doing and why, they are usually quite willing to wait a few months for their education. In 15 years at the Stanford Patient Education Research Center, we have had 4,000 people participate in randomized studies in which the controls have been asked to wait 4 to 8 months. We have seldom had any problems either getting or maintaining the control group.

If a randomized comparison group is not possible, then it may be possible to find a similar but nonrandomized comparison group. This could be hypertension patients from another hospital. Or you might want to give your program in one part of the city, using people in another part of the city as controls. In any case, the important thing to remember is that the comparison group must be as similar to the treatment group as possible.

The above discussion has been designed to give you a few ideas about the thought process that goes into any evaluation. You cannot become an evaluation expert overnight. Like anything else, evaluation is a skill. You need practice and guidance to become proficient. However, all practitioners can be good evaluators. Just do not be afraid to stick your toe into the water. You might even find that you like swimming!

¤ BIBLIOGRAPHY

Archer, A., & Fleshman, R. (Eds.). (1985). *Community health nursing patterns and practice.* Boston: Darbery.

Brown, R. A., & Beck, J. S. (1994). *Medical statistics on personal computers.* Plymouth, UK: BMJ.

DeVellis, R. F. (1991). *Scale development: Theory and applications.* Newbury Park, CA: Sage.

Green, L. W., & Lewis, F. M. (1986). *Measurement and evaluation in health education and health promotion.* Palo Alto, CA: Mayfield.

Kanji, G. K. (1993). *100 Statistical tests.* Menlo Park, CA: Sage.

Windsor, R. A., Barabowski, T., Clark, N., & Cutter, G. (1994). *Evaluation of health promotion and education programs* (2nd ed.). Palo Alto, CA: Mayfield.

Appendix 2A
Patient Education Evaluation Scales

This appendix consists of several self-administered question-naires that have been used in evaluating patient education programs. All of these scales have met all the standard criteria for questionnaires and have been published in national journals.

¤ VISUAL ANALOGUE SCALES

Below are sample visual analogue scales for pain and quality of life. Such scales are an excellent easy way to measure
subjective states.

Pain Visual Analogue Scale

We are interested in learning whether or not you are
affected by pain because of your illness. Please mark an X on
the line below to describe your arthritis pain in the *recent past.*

Pain as bad
as can be |————————————————| No pain
          SEVERE   MODERATE   SLIGHT

Quality of Life Visual Analogue Scale

Take a moment and think of the best possible life. Now, on
the line below, place an X to indicate where your life is *now.*

Worst   Best
possible |————————————————| possible
life   life

Scoring

Measure in centimeters with ruler, with 10 being "Pain as
bad as can be" or "Worst possible life" and 0 being "No pain"
or "Best possible life." Enter the number where the middle of
the X is located. Enter whole numbers, not decimals. If the X

is between centimeters, round down if below 0.5, and round up if 0.5 and above.

Note: The line must be *exactly* 10 cm long. When reproducing, make sure your printer or copy machine reproduces at exactly 100%. (Kodak copiers, for example, generally reproduce at 100%; Xerox copiers don't.) You cannot have a reliable measurement if the line isn't exactly the same length each time.

¤ BIBLIOGRAPHY

Dixon, J. S., & Bird, H. A. (1981). Reproducibility along a 10 cm vertical visual analogue scale. *Annals of the Rheumatic Diseases, 40,* 87-89.

Downie, W. W., Leatham, P. A., Rhind, V. A., Pickup, M. E., & Wright, V. (1978). The visual analogue scale in the assessment of grip strength. *Annals of the Rheumatic Diseases, 37,* 382-384.

Downie, W. W., Leatham, P. A., Rhind, V. A., Wright, V., Branco, J. A., & Anderson, J. A. (1978). Studies with pain rating scales. *Annals of the Rheumatic Diseases, 37,* 378-381.

Jacobsen, M. (1965). The use of rating scales in clinical research. *British Journal of Psychiatry, 3,* 545-546.

Scott, R. J., & Huskisson, E. C. (1976). Graphic representation of pain. *Pain, 2,* 175-184.

Scott, R. J., & Huskisson, E. C. (1977). Measurement of functional capacity with visual analogue scales. *Rheumatology and Rehabilitation, 16,* 257-259.

¤ HEALTH ASSESSMENT QUESTIONNAIRE

The Health Assessment Questionnaire measures disability. It has been used in the National Health Survey and in many chronic disease studies. One section, assessing disability, is reproduced here.

Name _____ Date _____

In this section we are interested in learning how your illness affects your ability to function in daily life. Please feel free to add any comments on the back of this page.

Please check the response which best describes your usual abilities OVER THE PAST WEEK:

	Without ANY Difficulty	*With SOME Difficulty*	*With MUCH Difficulty*	*UNABLE to Do*
DRESSING & GROOMING Are you able to:				
—Dress yourself, including tying shoelaces and doing buttons?	_____	_____	_____	_____
—Shampoo your hair?	_____	_____	_____	_____
ARISING Are you able to:				
—Stand up from a straight chair?	_____	_____	_____	_____
—Get in and out of bed?	_____	_____	_____	_____
EATING Are you able to:				
—Cut your meat?	_____	_____	_____	_____
—Lift a full cup or glass to your mouth?	_____	_____	_____	_____
—Open a new milk carton?	_____	_____	_____	_____

WALKING
Are you able to:
—Walk outdoors on flat ground?   _____   _____   _____   _____
—Climb up five steps?   _____   _____   _____   _____

Please check any AIDS OR DEVICES that you usually use for
any of these activities:

_____ Cane   _____ Devices used for dressing
_____ Walker   (button hook, zipper pull,
_____ Crutches   long-handled shoe horn, etc.)
_____ Wheelchair   _____ Built-up or special utensils
_____ Special or built-   _____ Other (Specify: _____)
        up chair

Please check any categories for which you usually need HELP
FROM ANOTHER PERSON:

_____ Dressing and Grooming   _____ Eating
_____ Arising   _____ Walking

Please check the response which best describes your usual
abilities OVER THE PAST WEEK:

	Without ANY Difficulty	With SOME Difficulty	With MUCH Difficulty	UNABLE to Do
HYGIENE				
Are you able to:				
—Wash and dry your body?	_____	_____	_____	_____
—Take a tub bath?	_____	_____	_____	_____
—Get on and off the toilet?	_____	_____	_____	_____

Appendix 2A   51
REACH
Are you able to:
—Reach and get down a 5-pound
  object (such as a bag of sugar) from
  just above your head?   _____   _____   _____   _____
—Bend down to pick up clothing
  from the floor?   _____   _____   _____   _____

GRIP
Are you able to:
—Open car doors?   _____   _____   _____   _____
—Open jars which have been
  previously opened?   _____   _____   _____   _____
—Turn faucets on and off?   _____   _____   _____   _____

ACTIVITIES
Are you able to:
—Run errands and shop?   _____   _____   _____   _____
—Get in and out of a car?   _____   _____   _____   _____
—Do chores such as vacuuming
  or yardwork?   _____   _____   _____   _____

Please check any AIDS OR DEVICES that you usually use for
any of these activities:

_____ Raised toilet seat   _____ Long-handled appliances
_____ Bathtub seat   for reaching
_____ Jar opener (for jars   _____ Long-handled appliance
        previously opened)   in bathroom
_____ Bathtub bar   _____ Other (Specify: _____)

Please check any categories for which you usually need HELP
FROM ANOTHER PERSON:

_____ Hygiene   _____ Gripping and opening things
_____ Reaching   _____ Errands and chores

Administration of the Questionnaire

The HAQ is usually self-administered. The questionnaire is usually mailed to patients every 6 months and they are asked to complete it without additional instructions. Follow-up phone calls will sometimes have to be made regarding any missing or ambiguous responses. The HAQ can also be administered in a face-to-face or telephone interview format by trained outcome assessors.

Scoring of the HAQ Disability Index

General Description

This section is designed to assess the patient's functional ability over the past week. It is composed of eight categories, each of which has at least two component questions. Patients are also asked to indicate their use of any aids or devices or if they need help from another person for any of these activities.

Specifics

The eight categories are dressing & grooming, arising, eating, walking, hygiene, reach, grip, and activities. For each of these categories, patients are asked to record the amount of difficulty they may have in performing various activities. Do not define terms such as SOME, MUCH, or USUAL for the patients. Let them use their own frame of reference. For example, if you are asked what "SOME" means, you can say whatever you think of as "SOME."

The time frame for these questions is OVER THE PAST WEEK. Some patients question whether we are interested in a particularly good or bad time that is out of this time frame. We are not. Patients sometimes are concerned that we are missing those times when their functional ability changes. By repeating the questionnaire at specific time periods, we can look at the patterns of function. If we asked patients to complete this section only when they were feeling particularly good or bad, then we would be getting a false picture.

We are interested in the patients' USUAL abilities using their usual equipment. The score is not increased if the patients have difficulties sometimes or occasionally require help.

Patients sometimes wonder how to answer the questions for various reasons:

- If they don't do things out of preference (shampooing hair, taking a tub bath, keeping heavy objects above their heads), then they should leave them blank since we want to know what they can do.
- If they have adapted or modified things (clothing, faucets, cars), then they should answer the questions based on their usual equipment. If they have no difficulty using the adapted equipment, then they would mark the "no difficulty" column. The adapted equipment (aids and devices) will be taken into account in the assistance variables.
- If they can open their own car doors but not others, then they should respond considering their usual equipment and encounters.
- Patients should make their own decisions concerning distance in answering the question about walking.

Scoring and Coding DRESSNEW, RISENEW, EATNEW, WALKNEW, HYGNNEW, REACHNEW, GRIPNEW, ACTIVNEW

Possible responses for the component questions are:

Without ANY difficulty   = 0
With SOME difficulty   = 1
With MUCH difficulty   = 2
UNABLE to do   = 3

The highest score recorded by the patient for any component question determines the score for that category. If a component question is left blank or the response is too ambiguous to assign a score, then the score for that category is determined by the remaining completed question(s). If all component questions are blank or if more than one answer is given, then call the patient. If the patient's mark is between the response columns, then move it to the closest one. If it's directly between the two, move it to the higher one.

Record the 0 to 3 value for each of the categories directly on the questionnaire in the shaded area.

DRESSNEW—Dressing & grooming   HYGNNEW—Hygiene
RISENEW—Arising   REACHNEW—Reach
EATNEW—Eating   GRIPNEW—Grip
WALKNEW—Walking   ACTIVNEW—Activities

Scoring and Coding DRSGASST, RISEASST, EATASST, WALKASST, HYGNASST, RCHASST, GRIPASST, ACTVASST

All of the disability items on the HAQ have a companion variable that is used to record what type(s) of assistance, if any, the participant uses for his/her usual activities. These variables

(DRSGASST, RISEASST, EATASST, WALKASST, HYGNASST, RCHASST, GRIPASST, ACTVASST) are to be coded as follows:

0 = No assistance is needed.
1 = A special device is used by the patient in his/her usual activities.
2 = The patient usually needs help from another person.
3 = The patient usually needs BOTH a special device AND help from another person.

Devices associated with each category:

DRESSING & GROOMING	Devices used for dressing (button hook, zipper pull, long-handled shoe horn, etc.)
ARISING	Built up or special chair
EATING	Built up or special utensils
WALKING	Cane, walker, crutches
HYGIENE	Raised toilet seat, bathtub seat, bathtub bar, long-handled appliances in bathroom
REACH	Long-handled appliances for reach
GRIP	Jar opener (for jars previously opened)

Note that this assignment of devices to particular disability categories assumes that the devices are used only for the purpose for which they are designed. For example, we assume that if a participant indicates that he/she uses a cane, he/she uses the cane as an aid in walking. However, it is possible for the patient to use that cane as an aid in performing other activities. For example, the patient may check off the cane listed at the bottom of page 1 of the HAQ (or wrote "cane" under the "other" slot) and then write a little note in the margin stating that the cane is also used on a regular basis as an aid in helping himself/herself to rise out of a chair and to rise off of the toilet. In such a case, the WALKASST, RISEASST, and HYGNASST variables should be coded as "1" to reflect the patient's use of a cane in these three areas of daily functioning. If you are unsure whether the patient is using one of the devices specified above for the purpose for which it is designed, call the patient to ask him/her exactly what are the activities for which he/she uses it.

Devices written in the "Other" sections or notes written next to any component questions are considered if they would be used for any of the stated categories. Permanent adaptations of the person's environment (e.g., changing faucets in the bathroom or kitchen, using velcro closures on clothing) should also be counted as aids and devices.

Computed Variables

The scoring variables and scoring rules allow the computation of two disability indices.

For the *Standard Disability Index,* a new set of component scores are computed by adjusting the score for each component, if necessary, based on the participant's use of an aid or device or assistance for that component. If either devices and/ or help from another person is checked for a category, the score is set to "2," unless the score is already "3" (i.e., scores of "0" or "1" are increased to "2"). For example, if the highest score for the dressing component is "1" and the patient says he or she uses a device for dressing, the computed component score would be "2." The sum of the computed component scores is then calculated and divided by the number of categories answered. This gives a score in the 0 to 3.0 range. The disability index is not computed if the patient does not have scores for at least 6 categories.

The *Alternative Disability Index* is calculated by adding the scores for each of the categories using the new component variables and dividing by the number of categories answered. This gives a score in the 0 to 3.0 range. The assistance variables are not used to calculate the alternative disability index. The disability index is not computed if the patient does not have scores for at least 6 categories.

SOURCE: From "Measurement of Patient Outcome in Arthritis," by J. F. Fries, R. G. Kraines, and H. R. Holman, 1980, *Arthritis and Rheumatism, 23,* pp. 137-145. Copyright 1980 by James F. Fries. Reprinted with permission.

¤ THE CENTER FOR EPIDEMIOLOGIC
STUDIES DEPRESSION SCALE (CES-D)

The Center for Epidemiologic Studies Depression Scale (CES-D; Radloff, 1977) was developed to measure depression in the general population. We like it better than other self-administered depression scales because it is especially sensitive in picking up subclinical depression. This level of depression is very common in people suffering from physical disease.

Below is a list of some of the ways you may have felt or behaved. Please indicate how often you have felt this way during the *past week* by checking the appropriate space.

	Rarely or None of the Time (Less Than 1 Day)	Some or a Little of the Time (1-2 Days)	Occasionally or a Moderate Amount of Time (3-4 Days)	All of the Time (5-7 Days)
1. I was bothered by things that usually don't bother me.				
2. I did not feel like eating; my appetite was poor.				
3. I felt that I could not shake off the blues, even with help from my family.				
4. I felt that I was just as good as other people.				
5. I had trouble keeping my mind on what I was doing.				
6. I felt depressed.				
7. I felt that everything I did was an effort.				
8. I felt hopeful about the future.				
9. I thought my life had been a failure.				
10. I felt fearful.				

11. My sleep was restless.	_____	_____	_____	_____
12. I was happy.	_____	_____	_____	_____
13. I talked less than usual.	_____	_____	_____	_____
14. I felt lonely.	_____	_____	_____	_____
15. People were unfriendly.	_____	_____	_____	_____
16. I enjoyed life.	_____	_____	_____	_____
17. I had crying spells.	_____	_____	_____	_____
18. I felt sad.	_____	_____	_____	_____
19. I felt that people disliked me.	_____	_____	_____	_____
20. I could not get going.	_____	_____	_____	_____

Scoring

	Item Weights			
	Rarely or None of the Time (Less Than 1 Day)	*Some or a Little of the Time (1-2 Days)*	*Occasionally or a Moderate Amount of Time (3-4 Days)*	*All of the Time (5-7 Days)*
1. I was bothered by things that usually don't bother me.	0	1	2	3
2. I did not feel like eating; my appetite was poor.	0	1	2	3
3. I felt that I could not shake off the blues, even with help from my family.	0	1	2	3
4. I felt that I was just as good as other people.	3	2	1	0
5. I had trouble keeping my mind on what I was doing.	0	1	2	3
6. I felt depressed.	0	1	2	3
7. I felt that everything I did was an effort.	0	1	2	3
8. I felt hopeful about the future.	3	2	1	0
9. I thought my life had been a failure.	0	1	2	3
10. I felt fearful.	0	1	2	3

11. My sleep was restless.	0	1	2	3
12. I was happy.	3	2	1	0
13. I talked less than usual.	0	1	2	3
14. I felt lonely.	0	1	2	3
15. People were unfriendly.	0	1	2	3
16. I enjoyed life.	3	2	1	0
17. I had crying spells.	0	1	2	3
18. I felt sad.	0	1	2	3
19. I felt that people disliked me.	0	1	2	3
20. I could not get going.	0	1	2	3

The score is the sum of the 20 item weights. Possible range is 0 to 60. If more than four questions are missing answers, do not score the CES-D. A person with a score of 16 or more is considered depressed.

¤ BIBLIOGRAPHY

Radloff, L. S. (1977). The CES-D scale: A self-report depression scale for research in the general population. *Applied Psychological Measurement, 1,* 385-401.

¤ SELF-REPORTED MEDICATION-TAKING SCALE

The Self-Reported Medication-Taking Scale is a quick, easy way to measure compliance. It was designed for a high-blood-pressure study. Although other means of monitoring compliance, such as laboratory testing, may produce more accurate results, this scale should not be discounted. It does quite well in giving a general idea of what is happening.

	(Circle *one*)	
1. Do you ever forget to take your medicine?	Yes	No
2. Are you careless at times about taking your medicine?	Yes	No
3. When you feel better, do you sometimes stop taking your medicine?	Yes	No
4. Sometimes if you feel worse when you take the medicine, do you stop taking it?	Yes	No

Scoring

To score, code Yes = 0, No = 1. The sum of the answers is the score. A score of 4 is considered high compliance, 3 is moderate compliance, and 2 or less is low compliance.

SOURCE: From "Concurrent and Predictive Validity of a Self-Reported Measure of Medication Adherence," by D. E. Morisky, L. W. Green, and D. M. Levine, 1986, *Medical Care, 24,* pp. 67-74. Copyright 1986 by J. B. Lippincott Company. Reprinted with permission.

¤ GROUP HEALTH ASSOCIATION OF AMERICA CONSUMER SATISFACTION SURVEY

This survey is a means of measuring patient satisfaction.

Your Health Care

Thinking about *your own health care,* how would you rate the following?

(Circle one number on each line)

	Poor	Fair	Good	Very Good	Excellent
OVERALL					
1. Overall, how would you evaluate health care at [plan]?	1	2	3	4	5
ACCESS: Arranging for and Getting Care					
2. Convenience of location of the doctor's office	1	2	3	4	5
3. Hours when the doctor's office is open	1	2	3	4	5
4. Access to specialty care if you need it	1	2	3	4	5
5. Access to hospital care if you need it	1	2	3	4	5
6. Access to medical care in an emergency	1	2	3	4	5
7. Arrangements for making appointments for medical care by phone	1	2	3	4	5
8. Length of time spent waiting at the office to see the doctor	1	2	3	4	5
9. Length of time you wait between making an appointment for routine care and the day of your visit	1	2	3	4	5

10. Availability of medical information or advice by phone	1	2	3	4	5
11. Access to medical care whenever you need it	1	2	3	4	5
12. Services available for getting prescriptions filled	1	2	3	4	5

FINANCES

13. Protection you have against hardship due to medical expenses	1	2	3	4	5
14. Arrangements for you to get the medical care you need without financial problems	1	2	3	4	5

TECHNICAL QUALITY

15. Thoroughness of examinations and accuracy of diagnoses	1	2	3	4	5
16. Skill, experience, and training of doctors	1	2	3	4	5
17. Thoroughness of treatment	1	2	3	4	5

COMMUNICATION

18. Explanations of medical procedures and tests	1	2	3	4	5
19. Attention given to what you have to say	1	2	3	4	5
20. Advice you get about ways to avoid illness and stay healthy	1	2	3	4	5

CHOICE AND CONTINUITY

21. Number of doctors you have to choose from	1	2	3	4	5
22. Arrangements for choosing a personal doctor	1	2	3	4	5
23. Ease of seeing the doctor of your choice	1	2	3	4	5

INTERPERSONAL CARE

24. Friendliness and courtesy shown to you by your doctors	1	2	3	4	5
25. Personal interest in you and your medical problems	1	2	3	4	5

26. Respect shown to you, attention to your privacy	1	2	3	4	5
27. Reassurance and support offered to you by your doctors and staff	1	2	3	4	5
28. Friendliness and courtesy shown to you by staff	1	2	3	4	5
29. Amount of time you have with doctors and staff during a visit	1	2	3	4	5

OUTCOMES

30. The outcomes of your medical care, how much you are helped	1	2	3	4	5
31. Overall quality of care and services	1	2	3	4	5

Attitudes Toward Care

Below are some things people say about their medical care. Please read each one carefully, keeping in mind your health care plan. Although the statements may look similar, please answer each one separately.

(Circle one number on each line)

	Strongly Agree	Agree	Not Sure	Disagree	Strongly Disagree
32. I am very satisfied with the medical care I receive	1	2	3	4	5
33. There are some things about the medical care I receive that could be better	1	2	3	4	5
34. The medical care I have been receiving is just about perfect	1	2	3	4	5
35. I am dissatisfied with some things about the medical care I receive	1	2	3	4	5

Scoring

For all items except 32 through 34:
1 = poor
2 = fair
3 = good
4 = very good
5 = excellent

For items 32 through 34, score as follows:
1 = 5
2 = 4
3 = 3
4 = 2
5 = 1

All items and scales are scored by the above scoring, with the higher ratings being best.

You have a choice of using the scores for the individual items or clustering items (as they are on the questionnaire) into a scale (Access, Finances, Technical Quality, Communication, Choice and Continuity, Interpersonal Care, Outcomes, and Attitudes Toward Care). To score a scale, add the score of all the items and divide by the number of items in the scale. This will give you the mean or average scale score.

If half or more of the items are missing, consider the whole scale as missing. Do not count missing items when you are figuring a scale score.

Please note: The complete Consumer Satisfaction Survey contains a number of additional scales for rating one's health insurance plan.

SOURCE: From *GHAA's Consumer Satisfaction Survey and User's Manual* (2nd ed.), by A. R. Davies and J. E. Ware, 1991, Washington, DC: Group Health Association of America, Inc. Copyright 1991 by the Group Health Association of America, Inc. Reprinted with permission.

How Do I Get From a Needs Assessment to a Program?
Program Planning and Implementation

Kate Lorig

Putting together a patient education program is a little like being a juggler. You have to keep several balls in the air at the same time. The first ball is nearly always a needs assessment; the other balls are launched more or less simultaneously. At the same time that you are considering how to evaluate your program, you should be launching the plan for its implementation. In other words, you will have to make many decisions about what your program will look like.

¤ SETTING PRIORITIES: CHOOSING WHAT TO TEACH IN THE TIME ALLOTTED

Whether patient education is given in 5-, 10-, or 15-minute blocks or several hour-long classes, you never have enough time to teach everything. Thus it is necessary to set priorities. Making decisions about what to teach requires three steps:

1. Listing all behaviors affecting the particular condition
2. Determining which behaviors are most important in affecting health status
3. Determining which behaviors are the easiest to change, given a limited amount of educational time

Let us examine these three steps.

Listing Behaviors

For all health conditions there are a number of behaviors that, if changed, would affect the condition. For example, someone with hypertension might be advised to stop smoking, lose weight, cut down on sodium, exercise, reduce stress, and comply with medication usage. A similar list can be made for any condition. The first step in setting priorities is to make a list of all behaviors that might affect the condition.

Determining the Effect of Each Behavior

This is probably the most difficult part of priority setting. As health educators, we do not know a great deal about the relative effects of health behaviors on health outcomes. However, not all behaviors are equal. In lowering blood pressure, medication compliance and smoking cessation are probably the most important, with weight loss, sodium reduction, and exercise coming somewhere in the middle. Stress reduction, although very popular, probably has only a limited long-term effect on hypertension. Therefore, in choosing priority behaviors, you should first look at smoking cessation and medication compliance.

The question arises: How do you determine the relative effects? This is where you should use experts. Ask physicians or epidemiologists to help with this problem. You can also read the studies yourself. One important note of caution: Do not set priorities based on the popular press. For example, recently we have been urged to cut down on dietary cholesterol. There is no question that blood cholesterol affects heart disease and that for someone with very high blood cholesterol, cutting down on dietary cholesterol may help. However, big changes in blood cholesterol usually require medication. Most of the major studies showing that lowering cholesterol has reduced heart disease have accomplished this primarily through medication usage. Our knowledge of the effects of lowering cholesterol through dietary means is much more fragmentary. This is especially true for the elderly. What does all this mean? Should we do nothing? No, we should continue to urge a low-cholesterol diet, but also realize that this should not be at a cost of quality of life. The fad of today may well be seen as the mistake of tomorrow. Remember, 30 years ago we were urging everyone to eat red meat. In short, be responsible for knowing a little about the research base for behaviors that you are urging others to change.

Determining Which Behaviors Are Relatively Easy to Change

We all know that some behaviors are easier to change than others. For example, it is relatively easy to get someone to take a pill once a day and much more complex to get someone to bring and keep his or her weight down. The next step is to look at the items you listed as important to health and rank how easy or difficult each is to change. One quick and not always accurate rule of thumb is that it is usually easier to get people to add behaviors than to give up behaviors. Depending on the amount of time, you can now choose which behaviors are most appropriate for your program. If you have only 10 minutes with a hypertensive patient, you might concentrate on medication compliance and lowering sodium intake. On the other hand, if you have 10 hours, you might work on diet, exercise, and smoking behaviors in addition to compliance and sodium reduction.

Another way of setting priorities is to let patients choose. Make a list of all the things that someone might do. For example, the list for losing weight might include not eating after 7 p.m., not eating between meals, broiling foods instead of frying them, cutting down on sweets, cutting down on fats, eating more fruit and vegetables, and increasing exercise. Then let patients choose the behaviors that they feel they can accomplish. This method has two advantages. First, you do not have to tell patients everything about dieting and exercise. If there is something on the list they do not understand, they can ask. Second, patients are given choices and control. The more the new health behaviors are chosen rather than prescribed, the better the chance that they will be adopted.

In short, priority setting is based on the amount of time, the importance of the behavior, and the ease with which the behavior can be changed.

¤ REFINING YOUR CONTENT

Once you have decided on your target behaviors, the next step is to define what someone needs to know and what skills he or she must have to accomplish the behaviors. For example, patients with hypertension probably do not need to know the anatomy and physiology of the cardiovascular system. However, they do need to know the most effective ways to stop smoking and to remain nonsmokers. They need skills in fending off the social pressures to overeat and smoke, and they need to know how to change the environmental cues for smoking and eating. One of the greatest errors in many patient education programs is to spend a lot of time on interesting "facts" at the expense of learning and practicing necessary skills.

Sometimes refining content is almost self-evident. To comply with appropriate medication use, patients must know when to take the medication and how much to take. Often, to learn about necessary skills and knowledge, it is necessary to know the literature. In many areas of patient education, including smoking cessation, dietary changes, and exercise programs, there has been research on what patients need to know and do. You may have to juggle, but you don't have to recreate the whole circus.

¤ SETTING OBJECTIVES

Once you have done your needs assessment and chosen your content, the next step is to write objectives. These objectives make clear what you are trying to accomplish and will serve as standards for evaluation. Just as there are two types of evaluations, there are two types of objectives.

Process objectives are those by which you determine the process of the patient education. Examples are:

- Fifty people will receive diabetes education this year.
- Publicity for the program will appear in six newsletters.
- Each participant will speak at least once at each session.
- Some 70% of the participants will make a contract for at least one behavior change.

Notice that in writing process objectives, we have said nothing about changing health behaviors or health status. Instead, we have dealt with managerial and teaching process.

Outcome objectives tell what we hope to accomplish in terms of changes in health behavior or health status. Examples are:

- After 2 hours of instruction, 70% of the diabetics will be able to self-inject insulin.
- By the end of the course, 80% of the participants will report that they walk four or more blocks three times a week.
- After instruction, 60% of the patients will have a diastolic blood pressure below 90.
- Sixty percent of the persons screened at the health fair and found to have a high cholesterol reading will see a doctor within 1 month.

How to Write Objectives

All objectives have three parts: (a) an action, (b) criteria for the action, and (c) criteria for judging if the action has been accomplished.

An Action

The action or verb part of the objective must be something that you can hear or see. Sometimes you can also use smelling or tasting verbs. However, these are not always useful in patient education objectives. *Report, eat, walk,* and *have a diastolic pressure* are good action words for an objective. On the other hand, *know, understand, think,* and *feel* are not good action words. There is no way that you can see someone "knowing." If your objective is that the participants will have more knowledge, then the objective should read, "Eighty percent of the participants will score 70 or above on a diabetes quiz" or "When asked to name their medications, 75% of the participants will be able to name all the prescription medication that they will be taking when they leave the hospital." "Participants will feel more in control of their asthma" is not a good objective. A better one is "Eighty percent of the patients will increase their score by 10 or more points on an asthma self-efficacy scale."

Probably the most important part of writing an objective is choosing the correct action. The question to ask yourself is "Who cares?" It is all fine and good that patients score well on a quiz. However, we know that changes in knowledge do not necessarily lead to changes in behavior or health status. If they did we would have no smokers, alcoholics, overweight people, or people who do not floss their teeth. Thus knowledge objectives are probably not the best for most patient education programs. Instead, write objectives about what you want patients to accomplish by lowering cholesterol or blood pressure, stopping smoking, taking medications as directed, or following an exercise program. If the outcome does not make a difference, then it probably should not be included as an objective. Rereading the first part of this chapter on choosing content should help you in forming your objectives.

Criteria for the Action

This part of the objective answers the questions *who, what, when,* and *where:* for example, "after the course," "the participants," "the siblings of burn patients," "cholesterol or blood pressure reading," "given a choice of cooking oils." If you do not know who is going to do something, and how, when, or where people are going to do it, then there is no way of judging if it happens.

Criteria for Judging If the Action Happens

This part of the objective answers the question of *how many* or *how much.* It almost always deals with numbers: for example, "80% of the participants," "diastolic blood pressure of 90 or below," "increase at least 10 points," "four blocks, three times a week." Without this criterion, you have no way of knowing if you reached your objective. It is fine to say that patients will lower their blood pressure. However, you also need to know how many participants lower their blood pressure and by how much. Is a program successful if 2 out of 100 patients accomplish what you want them to accomplish? Probably not.

Objectives and Program Planning

Let us now look at how objectives can be applied to program planning. First, you should write only a few (fewer than 10) overall objectives for your program. These program objectives also form the basis for your outcome evaluation (see Chapter 2, the section "Outcome or Summative Evaluation"). Then write objectives for each session or patient encounter. For example, the overall objective for a hypertension course might be "At the end of the course, 70% of the participants will have a diastolic pressure below 90." The objectives for Session 1 of a hypertension course might be "Participants will (a) discuss three ways of lowering blood pressure and (b) choose one behavior they will change in the coming week."

In addition, process objectives should be written. These can usually be standardized for the entire intervention and do not need to be written for each session. An example is:

> Instructors will (a) take attendance at every class, (b) ensure that all participants say something at every session, (c) rein- force verbally or nonverbally (with nods of head, etc.) every person in every class, (d) ensure that 80% of the participants make a commitment to some activity at the end of Sessions 2 through 6, and (e) use brainstorming as a problem-solving technique.

Such process objectives form the basis for your process evalu- ation (see Chapter 2, the section "Process or Formative Evalu- ations").

In summary, objectives tell you where you are going and how you are going to get there. Writing them may seem bur- densome. However, the very process of writing process and outcome objectives forces you to clarify your thinking. More important, writing objectives enables you to communicate what you are thinking to others. Finally, objectives give you stand- ards by which to evaluate your program.

¤ PROCESS

By now you have chosen your content and written your objectives. The next step is to plan your process, or how you are going to teach. In achieving behavior change and changes in health status, process is at least as important as content and probably more important. As a general rule of thumb, it is a good idea to use several different processes each session. Also, the more interactive and participatory processes are, the more likely it is that change will occur. This section discusses a number of commonly used methods of patient education.

Media

Many people think of pamphlets or videotapes when they think of patient education. It is true that materials and media are very useful. However, seldom do they constitute a complete patient education program. Very few materials stand alone. Choosing and using materials is such a large topic that it is discussed in its own chapter (Chapter 4).

Mass Media

Mass media can take many forms, each with its own advantages and disadvantages. For example, newspaper, radio, and TV can reach large numbers of people and are excellent for making the public aware of a single need or event. It would not make much sense to use a small-group or even a lecture format to try to inform people about an impending flood. On the other hand, mass media messages are very expensive unless you use free public service announcements. The problem with free media is that you have no control over when your message will be released or sometimes the exact content of the message. To get good free use of the media requires a lot of press cultivation. Mass media messages, unless you can obtain a huge amount of media time and the message is very simple, are not good at changing health behaviors. Remember, stopping smoking is much more complicated than changing brands of detergent.

Local Media

Local media are an often overlooked form of media that in most communities is free for public access. Although it is true that local stations sometimes do not have a big audience, they can be used in some creative ways. For example, the Stanford Heart Disease Prevention Project produced a group of smoking-cessation programs. The programs used a lecture/discussion format, with a local media personality going through the program on TV. People were urged to watch individually or in small groups. There was a great deal of advance publicity to let people know about the coming programs. However, this was still a targeted audience of several thousand people. Of course, if you use local media, production time and skills will be fairly complex. Nevertheless, these can often be donated by students and others. A final advantage to the use of local media is that, if skillful, it can combine the advantages of mass media and small groups.

Computer-Based Education (CBE)

Computers are now becoming widely available in schools, libraries, and some homes. They are a much underutilized medium for health education. The advantage of computer-based education (CBE) is that it can reach a large audience. For example, there are programs on stress management, weight loss, and arthritis. These programs can be placed in schools and workplaces, as well as in health care settings. CBE can be somewhat individually tailored and can be paced to the needs of the individual. Once produced, it is relatively inexpensive. The disadvantage is that, as with any health education materials, good production requires both educational and technical skills. Also, CBE software must have compatible computers on which to run. With the advent of the Internet, the future will hold many new ways of using the computer for support groups and other patient education activities.

Films and Videotapes

Films and videotapes are excellent if you know exactly why you are using any one in particular. Videos allow you to illustrate something, sometimes in a more entertaining way than you could in an ordinary educational setting. In addition, they can illustrate some skills that are more difficult to show in a class setting, such as exercise or food preparation. If patients have VCRs, videotapes can be taken home to reinforce new behaviors. This is especially true for exercise programs. Finally, videotapes may be a means of providing education for patients with relatively rare diseases or with low reading skills.

One last note: Audiotapes are much easier and less expensive to produce than videotapes. They can sometimes be an excellent substitute for videotapes.

Group Processes

Brainstorming

This is one of the most common ways of gaining group participation in a nonthreatening manner. In addition to gaining participation, brainstorming is useful for creating many ideas and forming new ideas. Although it is often used, brainstorming is at times done incorrectly. Proper brainstorming consists of five steps.

1. Give participants directions—for example:

   I will ask you a question, and then you should give as many ideas as you can. Do not worry if the ideas sound silly or are a little strange. If you do not understand what someone else says, do not worry; we will talk about this later. Right now, all I want is for you to give as many ideas as you can.

2. Ask the question. It is important that you ask the question properly. To do this, it is best to write out the question before you begin your teaching. Do not say, "Give me some ideas about problems with medications"; rather, say, "What are some of the reasons that people do not take medications as prescribed by their doctor?" The first question is too vague and will result in all kinds of strange answers, whereas the second question is geared specifically to finding out why people do not comply with medication regimes.

3. Write down whatever the members of the group say. Keep writing items until no more are generated. Do not stop to discuss items. Just clarify that you are writing down what the participants say. It is useful to have two people conducting a brainstorm. One monitors the group for responses while the other writes. If you are the only trainer, you might ask someone in the group to write for you. However, be sure that the person writes what is actually said, not his or her interpretation. The list of ideas will be easier to read if you use two different colors and alternate the colors of the responses.

4. Ask if anyone needs clarification on what any of the items means. Have the person originally offering the item give the clarification.

5. Once all the items have been clarified, you can use the brainstorm material to summarize a point, begin a problem-solving session, or go on to further teaching or discussion. For exam-

ple, say you want to emphasize the advantages of exercise. Instead of giving a lecture, have the participants brainstorm all the advantages. Then you can correct any misconceptions or add the one or two things the group forgot. Another use of brainstorms is to solve problems. Someone in the group has a problem, such as not being able to avoid all the tempting food brought to work by coworkers. Instead of offering solutions yourself, ask the group for solutions. Then have the person with the problem indicate the one or two solutions he or she will try.

Role Playing

There are at least two reasons for using role playing in patient education. First, it allows participants to discuss issues that they might otherwise feel were too sensitive. Second, it allows participants to practice a new skill or rehearse for a future difficult situation. It should be noted that role playing is a difficult training skill and should be used only by a patient educator who is comfortable with the technique. Also, participants often feel threatened and therefore do not like to role-play. No one likes to be on display, especially if he or she might be made to look foolish. Several variations of role playing can help to control the situation and protect the participants.

Coaching. Give the participants a situation: For example, pretend that you are expressing dissatisfaction to your doctor. One person plays the doctor and one the patient. After the patient has expressed dissatisfaction, make some suggestion about how he or she might have done this differently, and then reenact the role play using your alternative. A variation on this is to ask members of the group for suggestions on how they might change the interaction. Again, it is important that the "patient" practice whatever solution is chosen. A second variation is to role-play in threes. The first person is the doctor, the second the patient, and the third the coach. In this case, have three situations so that everyone has a chance to play each role.

In a third variation, the patient educator takes one of the roles. For example, if a participant expresses difficulty in communicating with her child, the trainer takes the role of the child. In this way, the trainer can be sure that the responses are not too bizarre or threatening to the participant.

Group Role Plays. Here the trainer plays one role—for example, a patient who is very concerned about surgery—and the whole group plays the second role—for example, the nurse. First, one person counsels the "patient," and if he or she gets stuck, then someone else in the group takes over. This is a very non-threatening form of role playing and is easily controlled by the trainer.

Rehearsal. This is one of the most useful forms of role play. Give the patient a situation that he or she might encounter: For example, a postcardiac patient on a low-calorie diet goes out to eat with friends who urge her to have dessert. The patient can then practice refusal skills. People who rehearse difficult situations before actually encountering them do better when faced with them in the real world. By the way, rehearsal can easily be combined with coaching or group role plays.

Questioning

This is one of the most important of all patient education skills. Not only does it enable you to find out what the patient knows, but it can also be a useful way of teaching new skills. A basic rule for all questioning is that you should very seldom ask questions that can be answered by a "yes" or "no." Open-ended questions are much better. Do not ask, "Are you feeling better today?" Ask, "How are you feeling today?"

The following are some ways you might use questioning in your patient teaching:

- *The patient knows what he or she should do but is not doing it.* Ask, "Why do you smoke?" "What are you afraid might happen if you lost weight?" "What problems do you think you might have in starting an exercise program?"
- *You are helping a patient solve a problem.* Ask, "What solutions do you see for this problem?" "Where might you go to get other ideas?" "Which of these solutions would you like to try?" It is always better to teach problem-solving skills than to solve problems. Of course, in some situations, it is best to give an answer. If a patient asks which type of oil is low in cholesterol, there is no reason to cause frustration by telling him or her to go to the library.

One word of caution about questioning: Keep your voice tone neutral. Sometimes, when poorly asked, questions become judgmental—for example, "*Why* do *you* smoke?" instead of "*Why do you smoke?*"

Appendix 3A at the end of this chapter contains a list of questions from this book that you can ask patients to determine their needs, abilities, beliefs, and understanding.

Self-Monitoring

One of the best ways to get people to change behaviors is to let them monitor their own experience. People have a difficult time denying their own evidence. On the more positive side, self-monitoring helps a person see his or her problems or progress. Examples of self-monitoring include keeping a food diary or keeping track of when headaches occur. This information can then be used as the basis for behavior change. Self-monitoring can also be used as feedback, such as weekly weigh-ins and keeping track of exercise progress. This is like the feedback that is so important for obtaining skills mastery. For more on self-monitoring and skills mastery, see Chapter 9's section "Skills Mastery."

Creative patient educators can almost always build some self-monitoring techniques into their programs. The following are some concrete examples.

Diet

In many cases, patients are trying to change their diet—to lose weight, to lower cholesterol, to increase calcium, to decrease fats, or to conform to some regime such as a diabetic diet. In all these cases, a good place to start is to have patients keep a 4-day diet history in which they write down everything they eat as they eat it. The 4 days should probably be two weekend days and two weekdays. Fridays are more like weekend days than weekdays and thus should probably not be counted in the 4 days. This self-monitoring of food intake helps patients see where the problems lie and make plans to change. After being on a program for a while, they can again do a 4-day diary to see progress and check for any new problems.

Exercise

There are several ways to monitor exercise. The time spent exercising, the distance covered, the weights lifted, and the number of repetitions all help people see how they are progressing. While exercising, patients can take their own pulse to be sure that they are in an aerobic zone. A quick self-monitoring test is that if they cannot talk while exercising (unless, of course, they are swimming), then they are exercising too hard. Such simple self-monitoring guidelines are helpful in getting people started and take some of the fear away about doing too much.

Diabetes

Both urine testing and blood glucose monitoring are good ways of helping a diabetic self-monitor.

Hypertension

We know that many people have "white-coat hypertension," that is, their blood pressure is much higher in the doctor's office than at any other time. Therefore self-monitoring is very helpful. This can be done by getting patients to have their blood pressure taken regularly—perhaps at the supermarket that has a blood pressure machine, at community health centers, at the blood bank when giving blood, or at special health awareness weeks such as National Health Week. You might even teach clients how to take their own blood pressure and have equipment available at a convenient location. It is not important that the reading be 100% accurate. Rather, patients can see how their blood pressure changes over time. Of course, they need a little instruction in the meaning of the numbers.

Weight Loss

Scales are wonderful self-monitoring devices.

Asthma

In the case of asthma, you are trying to teach symptom recognition as well as to get people to act on their symptoms before they become serious. Peak-flow meters are useful for this. Monitoring can include keeping track of the number of times one must call the doctor, go into emergency, or miss work because of asthma. Also, patients can keep track of when medication is taken and its relationship to the seriousness of the attack. Most important, teach patients the early warning signs of an asthma attack so that with watchful monitoring, attacks can be averted.

There are no doubt hundreds of other ways to help people self-monitor. The more of these that you can build into the program, the more chance you will have of seeing real behavior change.

¤ WHO WILL TEACH THE PROGRAM?

It is usually best to decide who is going to present your program before it is developed. In this way you can include the presenters in program development. No one likes to be told to do something when he or she has had no input. But sometimes the program presenters are chosen only after the program is fully developed. This is especially true with very standardized programs.

¤ KNOWING WHAT TO TEACH
AND WHEN TO TEACH

Unfortunately, very few health professionals when working with patients one to one give much thought as to what they should teach. There is just no time. Therefore it is important that this decision process occur before the actual patient encounter. Thus, if a patient is in for bypass surgery, there should be a set protocol of things to teach. In fact, a checklist can be made up and then checked off as the patient education is delivered. The problem is not that professionals do not know the content. It is usually that they know too much and try to teach it all. Or they decide wisely that it is impossible to teach it all and therefore decide to teach nothing. In neither case are patient needs served. Again, what is needed is a priority-setting process that clarifies for all professionals what they should be teaching to any specific patient. Sometimes protocol or patient maps can be written that include what should be taught at each stage of the hospital stay: for example, preoperative, immediate postoperative, 2 or 3 days postoperative, and just before the patient leaves.

¤ KNOWING HOW TO TEACH

Most health professionals believe that they know how to teach. The reality is that most of us are only poor to fair patient educators. There are several reasons for this. First, few of us have had any formal training in patient education. Lacking this training, we try to emulate the teaching that we have received. The problem with this approach is that most school-type teaching is aimed at passing on knowledge. Patient education is aimed at changing behaviors or health status. Thus the teaching methods are different and must be learned and practiced.

In planning patient education programs, it is often necessary to teach patient education skills to the patient educators. These skills include the use of questioning, problem solving, goal setting, demonstration, and return demonstration. All of these are discussed earlier in this chapter or in Chapter 8 (see discussion of Figure 8.1, Questions 3 and 4). The important thing to note is that sometimes preparing a program is not enough. Significant time and effort must be spent on preparing health professionals to take on the role of successful patient educators.

¤ ONE-ON-ONE EDUCATION

One-on-one education is the most common type of patient education. It is what doctors, nurses, and other health professionals do at the bedside or in the clinic. In one-on-one education, there are four major considerations: time, knowing what to teach, knowing how to teach, and documenting what has been taught.

Time is an especially valuable commodity for doctors and, to a slightly lesser extent, for other health care professionals. Most doctors have only 10 to 20 minutes in which to interact with a patient. Therefore any education must be very quick. Some have called these 30-second interventions. So what can you do in 30 seconds? A great deal. A doctor can tell a patient, "I want you to stop smoking." This is one of the most powerful things a doctor can do to get someone to stop smoking. When doing a breast examination, the doctor can ask the patient to demonstrate how she examines her breasts. It has been found that getting a woman to touch her own breast is one of the best ways of ensuring future breast self-examination. Patients receiving prescriptions should always be asked how they are going to take the medication. This simple question helps to reveal any problems or misunderstandings. For example, one patient I know, when given an antibiotic labeled "Avoid exposure to sunlight," was very careful to keep the pills in a dark place. She never considered that she should avoid exposure to sun. Finally, the doctor can make referrals: "I know that you want to lose weight; here is a list of resources in our community to help you with that effort." These are just a few of the many possible 30-second interventions. In planning what you want doctors to do, it is important to be realistic.

Nurses, physiotherapists, occupational therapists, and other health professionals also have limited time. However, it may not be as limited as that of a doctor. Therefore you might think of 3- to 5-minute interventions that can realistically take place in the context of normal practice. If you use some of the priority-setting techniques discussed earlier in this chapter, these few minutes can be well utilized. In all cases it is important to separate out what a patient wants and needs to know from what the health professional wants to teach. The priority should always be on the former. Sometimes a compromise can be reached. If the patient is concerned about fatigue, and you want to teach about diet, you can frame your teaching by explaining how fatigue is often due to poor diet and thus can be helped by your suggestions.

¤ GROUP EDUCATION

Everything that we have said about one-on-one education is also true for group education. The difference is that the patient educator must have a greater variety of skills. In addition to all the one-on-one skills mentioned above, the educator, if he or she is going to do more than just lecture, must have skills in group process. Again, you are not born with these skills, but rather learn them from life experience or in a structured manner. A complete program for training patient educators is beyond the scope of this book. However, it is important to be aware of the possibility that you may need to train your patient educators or to see that they receive training.

¤ SPECIAL PROBLEMS WITH GROUPS

When patients come to groups, they come for different reasons and have different knowledge and skill levels. This is true no matter how specific you try to make your intake criteria. Therefore, in any group setting, meeting the needs of the individual members is a problem. There are several ways of handling this. First, make sure that all members know what to expect from the course. You can do this by using a matrix needs assessment (see Chapter 1). If you find that someone has needs that are very different from those of the rest of the group, you can let him or her know that this might not be the educational program for him or her. The outliers then have the option of staying or not. If they do stay, they will have no illusions about what the course will cover.

Another way of dealing with differences is to have everyone work on developing his or her own behavioral program. Thus, in a class on lowering cholesterol, some people may choose to increase fiber, others to cut down on eggs and dairy products, and still others to eat less red meat. When behaviors are flexible instead of prescriptive, they are much more likely to be meaningful (see section "Determining Which Behaviors Are Relatively Easy to Change" earlier in this chapter).

Finally, people with more knowledge and skills can be utilized to help those with less background. They can help in problem solving and can sometimes also be used as successful coping models (see Chapter 9 for a discussion of modeling). It is important that group education avoid being too rigid and prescriptive. If it is flexible, the varied backgrounds of the participants become an advantage, not a problem.

¤ PUTTING IT ALL TOGETHER

So far we have looked at many of the pieces that are necessary for putting together a patient education program. However, the real trick of patient education is putting the content and process together in a package that helps patients reach the outcome objectives. Such packaging usually takes the form of a protocol that outlines the general topics to be covered in the program. Good patient education protocols should also be so detailed that someone who is not familiar with the program can pick it up and replicate what you are doing. The reason such detailed protocols are not usually done is that they require considerable thought and preparation.

In preparing a protocol, there are several things to keep in mind.

1. *Write your objectives and be sure that what you are teaching is designed to meet these objectives.* For example, if you want a cardiac patient to exercise, do not spend the majority of your time explaining disease process. If you want an intervention to be interactive, use as little lecture as possible and build in interactive activities. These do not just happen; they have to be planned.

2. *Look at your resources—time, personal, money, space.* This will help you decide, if you are planning a one-on-one intervention, a mediated intervention (one that uses audio and/or visual materials), a one-time group meeting, a short course, or an ongoing support group. Do not assume that just because something has always been done one way it cannot be done another way. For example, people with knee pain usually have one-on-one appointments with physical therapists. In one major health facility, knee classes for people with knee pain are held twice weekly. People can attend as often as they wish. There is no waiting for appointments or concern because of insurance limits. Experience has shown that after initial hesitation, both patients and physical therapists are happy with the new system.

3. *Make sure that you vary your activities.* Everyone gets tired of the same format. Thus you might include some lecture, brainstorming, a film, and general discussion all in one session. It is especially important to encourage active participation of group members after lunch or dinner, as these are times that people sometimes get sluggish or are apt to fall asleep. A good time to introduce new activities is early in the day when people are fresh. Another trick of the trade is to save some of your most interesting material until last. This encourages people to stay to the end instead of leaving early.

4. *No matter what intervention you choose, do not waste the first few minutes.* This is the most important part of the intervention and the place where you can least afford mistakes. In educational terms, this is called the *set*. It (a) lets participants meet each other, (b) tells them what to expect, and (c) lets them decide to participate. Note how Activity 1 in the arthritis course protocol given in Appendix 3B at the end of this chapter was designed to meet these objectives. First, participants tell what arthritis means to them. This lets everyone know a little about

the others in the group. It also establishes the fact that there are common concerns. From a process point of view, it forces everyone to participate in a nonthreatening way. As the course is very interactive, it is important to model expectations early. It is one thing to tell participants that a class is interactive and quite another to see that interaction really happens.

After everyone participates, there is a brief lecture about expectations, and then participants are given an overview of the course and shown how their concerns are specifically met by this course.

Please note that the original request, "Write down and then share what arthritis means to you," is very specific. We do not ask people to "tell a little about themselves" or to talk about their arthritis. If either of these was used as an opener, people would give long discourses that would take up much more than the allotted time.

The opening is also kept on track by having the leaders model the desired behavior. The group will almost always follow the example of the first person. Therefore it is important to set a good example.

5. *If at all possible, build on activities over several weeks.* Thus, rather than having one session on diet and another on exercise, have two or more sessions that include and/or add to both of these subjects. In this way, participants will have a chance to go home, decide what they want to do, try things out, and report back with problems. Then there is still time to make changes.

6. *Try to use the same instructor or facilitator for every session.* This builds in continuity and helps to create rapport between the instructor and the participants, which is especially important for group education. If you use a different "expert" every

session, this is not patient education, but a lecture series; it is important to understand that it is very unlikely that such a series will result in behavior change. However, lecture series are usually very good for increasing knowledge.

7. *Consider using a* Sesame Street *approach.* Much of traditional patient education is taught by topic. In the first week we discuss exercise, in the next week nutrition, in the third week medications, and so on. No other education is carried out in this way. We usually have small doses of several topics, all of which are built on over time. This is what *Sesame Street* does. On each show there are several segments. Each segment is then built on each day. If you look at the topics discussed in the arthritis course protocol in Appendix 3B, you will see that exercise is discussed in four out of six sessions and that feedback and contracting are part of every session. All sessions discuss four or five topics. The advantage of this approach is that people are not overwhelmed with new material. They have a chance to try new activities, come back and make corrections, and then add to their program. The disadvantage is that you cannot have a different "expert" talk at each session.

8. *Use ritual.* There is security for both instructors and students in a known structure. This is one of the reasons that Alcoholics Anonymous and other 12-step programs are so successful. By ritual, we mean structure: Each class has a defined beginning, middle, and end that look much the same, session after session. In our arthritis protocol example (Appendix 3B), each class starts with feedback and ends with contracting. Structure helps to set group norms and expectations. It is one of the things that can be used to strengthen an intervention at no extra cost in time, money, or materials.

9. *Frame your teaching around patient needs and beliefs.* For example, topics could include pain management, dealing with anger, and beating fatigue rather than the use of medication,

coping, and exercise. Note that the same material is taught but in different ways. (For more about framing, see Chapter 4, "Does the Material Contain the Information the Patient Wants?")

10. *Do not try to change patient beliefs or practices unless they are causing harm.* If patients want to drink vinegar and honey, it probably will not hurt them. It is easier to add to beliefs than to change or destroy them.

11. *Be consistent with your messages.* If you are teaching self-management, then make patients responsible for finding information or making copies of materials. You cannot teach self-management and then manage for the patient.

12. *Remember that patients always have choices.* Often many activities will accomplish the same end. Patients always have the option of not doing what you suggest. There are two lessons here. First, do not be dogmatic. Second, remind patients that the decisions and choices are theirs.

13. *Do not try to crowd everything into whatever time you have.* The most common mistake in patient education is trying to include too much. In our need to give information, we often give up using the processes that make the information useful. Be very selective about what you teach. Everything that happens should be directly related to the objectives. You can always give your clients written material if they want more information.

(One important note: Patients will often ask many questions or become argumentative to avoid taking action. This is especially true in a class situation. To avoid this, tell the person that you will talk with him or her during break or after class.)

14. *Give attention for taking positive action.* All too often, we spend our time trying to convince people to do something they have no intention of doing. They like the attention they get for

not doing things. It is hard, but the best strategy is to help those who want help. For those who do not want to get down to business, remind them that it is their choice (see Number 9). When those who are hesitant to act see others who are successful, and when they do not get rewarded for inaction, there is a good chance that they will begin to manage their condition.

Appendix 3B at the end of this chapter comments on and reprints an actual protocol from a session of a patient education course (Lorig, 1990).

¤ DOCUMENTING WHAT YOU TEACH

There are at least two major reasons for documenting what you teach. First, in many areas, this is a requirement for hospital accreditation. More important, for programs to be successful, it is necessary to know what patients have been taught and what they still need to learn. If documentation is in place, a patient will not be taught about hypertension medications five times and never learn the importance of exercise.

Documentation can take many forms. If there is a set protocol, say a six-session diabetes course, then all you need to do is to document that a patient attended the course and that the protocol was delivered as written. Unfortunately, documentation is not always this easy. In one-on-one teaching, it is helpful to note in the chart what has been taught. The problem is that few people will go back through pages of chart notes to figure out what to teach next. Charting may be helpful for legal purposes but may not help the patient.

An alternative is to have a patient education page in the chart. This is easy to find and also serves as documentation. (See Chapter 10 for a sample documentation form.) The disadvantage is that it adds bulk to the chart. A variation of the patient education chart is a checklist of all the things that a patient should be taught about any set condition. Then when something is taught, the item can be checked off and initialed. This is even more effective if the checklist is kept on the patient's bed. In this case, anyone who does any education—nurses, physical therapists, occupational therapists, and doctors—can see what has already been done and what is left to do. This checklist can then be placed in the permanent chart when the patient goes home. Similar types of checklists can be kept in outpatient charts. In all cases, it is important to be clear on how the documentation will be used. There is no reason to go to all this trouble if the documentation has no meaning for the patient, for program planning, or as a legal or accreditation document.

¤ BIBLIOGRAPHY

Lorig, K. (1990). *Arthritis self-management leader's manual.* Atlanta, GA: Arthritis Foundation.

Mager, R. F. (1970). *Preparing instructional objectives.* Belmont, CA: Fearon.

Appendix 3A
Questions in Patient Education

Asking good questions is your best means of determining a patient's needs, abilities, beliefs, and understanding. It is a key to excellence in patient education.

In general, use open-ended questions to elicit a meaningful response; avoid questions that can be answered with "yes" or "no." Use a neutral, not judgmental, voice. For example:

Yes-No Question	*Open-Ended Question*
Are you feeling better today?	How are you feeling today?
Do you know why you should quit smoking?	Why do you smoke?
Are you going to start exercising?	What problems do you think you might have in starting an exercise program?
Can you cut back on meat?	What will be your biggest problem with cutting down on the amount of meat you are eating?
Do you have any questions?	What questions do you have?

The following is a list of additional questions from this book for your easy reference:

1. Questions on salient beliefs to give you insight into the patient's beliefs and concerns about a particular condition or behavior:
   - When you think of _____ (e.g., diabetes, exercise), what do you think of?
   - What would you do if _____?

2. Needs assessment questions to determine priorities for teaching:
   - What are your greatest problems in living with _____ (heart disease, a low-fat diet)?
   - Which changes would you like to start on? (give the patient a list of changes you are recommending, e.g., exercise, low-fat diet, quitting smoking, controlling stress, losing weight)
   - If you _____ (stop smoking, start exercising, etc.), what are you afraid might happen?
   - What do you think causes _____ (pain, diabetes, etc.)?
   - Why is exercise important to you?
   - Why don't you _____?

3. Questions to determine cultural issues that could affect health behavior:
   - What do you believe about your _____ (diabetes, stomach problem)?
   - What will make it better?
   - What do you expect me to do for you?

4. Questions to check for understanding (ask patients to repeat back what they understand):
   - So how much are you going to walk tomorrow after you are home?

5. Self-efficacy questions to determine likelihood of success:

- On a scale of 1 to 10, how sure are you that you can do
  _____ (a very specific behavior, such as walking for 15
  minutes 3 times a week)? (If patient's answer is 7 or less, ask
  him or her to revise his or her goal to ensure success.)

6. Questions to test the likelihood of compliance:

   - Do you think that it will help to (exercise, take medications)?

7. Questions to reinforce a new behavior:

   - Role play: "OK, say I'm your friend and you are you, and we
     are at a party and I am encouraging you to eat a piece of fried
     chicken. How would you say 'no thanks' to me?"

Appendix 3B
Protocol for a Session of the Arthritis Self-Help Course

The following is the protocol from the first 2-hour session of the Arthritis Self-Help Course. This patient education program is offered by the Arthritis Foundations of the United States and Australia, by the Arthritis Societies in Canada, and by Arthritis Care in Great Britain. The course is designed to be taught by a pair of leaders, at least one of whom is a layperson with arthritis. Self-efficacy theory serves as the theoretical framework for the course. As you read over this protocol, note that the session has specific objectives and that the activities are varied, starting with an interactive exercise. Activity 1 sets the tone for the following 12 hours. It clearly sets forth the expectations for the group's participation by reviewing the class guidelines (Chart 2). Also, within the first few minutes, there is a course overview (Chart 3) that helps participants decide if they have come to the right course.

Activity 2 reinforces this tone with a brief lecture on self-help principles.

Activity 3 is an example of helping participants to reinterpret physiological signs and symptoms. This is one of the ways to enhance self-efficacy (see Chapter 9, "Self-Efficacy Theory"). Note that this activity again is done in an interactive mode rather than lecture.

Activity 4 is a lecture on the disease process. These 15 minutes are the only ones during 12 hours of education devoted to disease process. Chart 4, as well as the other charts, is used to reinforce information that is given through lecture or other means.

Activity 5 is the first introduction to exercise. This topic is repeated and built upon during each of the following five sessions. Note that this activity uses both brainstorming and lecture.

Activity 6 is the ending for every class. Contracting is used to assist participants in gaining skills mastery. This is another important component for building self-efficacy. Note that this activity ends with a short visualization exercise to help participants fix in their minds both their contract and their success in accomplishing it.

In summary, this 2-hour session has used several educational processes, including the group's sharing of experience, lecture, visual charts, brainstorming, a short self-quiz, contracting, and visualization. In addition, it has covered several content areas, including a needs assessment, discussion of disease process, and introduction to exercise. In short, this first session sets the stage for the use of content and process for the entire 12 hours.

SESSION 1

Purpose:

1. To introduce the group members to each other
2. To inform the group about the general principles of self-help
3. To identify the group members' feelings about arthritis
4. To provide basic information about arthritis
5. To introduce group members to the importance of exercise

Objectives:

By the end of this session, the group members will be able to

1. State their role in the care of their arthritis
2. Define the differences between the major types of arthritis
3. State the benefits of physical fitness for arthritis
4. State the 3 parts of an exercise program
5. Make a contract for an arthritis-related behavior in the coming week

Materials:

1. Blank name tags for everyone
2. Easel
3. Blank flip charts/felt pens or blackboard chalk, prewritten Charts 1-5
4. *The Arthritis Helpbook* (Lorig & Fries, 1995) for each person
5. Pad of paper, extra pencils

***Plan Outline** (post this agenda at the beginning of class):*

Activity 1: Introduction (25 min.)

Activity 2: Overview of Self-Help Principles (10 min.)

Activity 3: Debunking Myths (10 min.)

Break (10 min.)

Activity 4: Introduction to Arthritis (15 min.)

Activity 5: Exercising for Fun and Fitness—Where to Start (20 min.)

Activity 6: Contracting (20 min.)

Activity 7: Closing (5 min.)

Activity 1: INTRODUCTION (25 min.)

Methods: Lecturette and group introductions
Note: Refer to Charts 1-3

Charts are shown throughout this manual with the material to be printed on the chart in bold CAPS (and the material you add verbally in parentheses).

1. As participants arrive, distribute name tags. Have them write the names they like to be called—large enough so that they can be read from across the room. Also, collect physician information forms (if necessary).
2. Welcome the group and introduce yourself, including the fact that you have arthritis (if true).
3. Group introduction. Have participants write down what arthritis means to them. Then have participants introduce themselves and share what arthritis means to them. One leader should list people's responses on the board or chart pad (Chart 1). Put a check mark next to a word or statement every time it is repeated by another person. Note: Save this chart (*Chart 1,*

Chart 1
WHAT ARTHRITIS MEANS TO ME

WHAT ARTHRITIS MEANS TO ME) to make comparisons of progress in the last session.

4. Describe the guidelines of the group. Refer to Chart 2.

Chart 2
GUIDELINES

1. **COME TO EVERY SESSION.**
2. **ASK ANYTHING YOU WANT.** (If we do not know the answer, we will get it. Also, if time is short, we may ask you to hold your questions for later.)
3. **DO YOUR HOMEWORK.** (It will not be graded but will make the course more valuable to you.)
4. **GIVE NEW ACTIVITIES AT LEAST A 2-WEEK TRIAL** (before deciding what will work best for you).
5. **MAKE AND COMPLETE A WEEKLY CONTRACT.**

---

5. Using Chart 3, give an overview of the course. Comment on how the content relates to "what arthritis means" to group members by referring back to their statements made at the beginning of the session (which you have on Chart 1).

6. If participants show an interest in topics that will not be addressed (such as surgery or research), state that they can probably find that information in *The Arthritis Helpbook*. If not, they can call the local Arthritis Foundation/Society.

Chart 3
COURSE OVERVIEW

Session 1: **Self-Help Principles**
Myths
Disease Process (OA/RA)
Exercise/Fitness
Feedback/Contracting

Session 2: **Flexibility/Strengthening Exercise**
Pain Management/Relaxation
Feedback/Contracting

Session 3: **Aerobic Exercise**
Depression
Distraction
Guided Imagery
Feedback/Contracting

Session 4: **Nutrition**
Osteoporosis
Nontraditional Treatments
Self-Talk
Problem-Solving
Feedback/Contracting

Session 5: **Communication Skills**
Working With Your Doctor
Fitness Progress
Visualization
Feedback/Contracting

Session 6: **Medications**
Fatigue
Sharing Accomplishments
Feedback/Contracting—Future Goals

Activity 2: OVERVIEW OF SELF-HELP PRINCIPLES (10 min.)

Introduction to the participative nature of this course
Method: Lecturette

1. Although the cure for arthritis is unknown, there are a variety of known treatments to *control* arthritis (i.e., to relieve discomfort and reduce disability). It is your responsibility to learn as much as possible about these treatments.
2. *Self-help* means being willing to learn about and assume responsibility for the daily care of your arthritis.
3. The Arthritis Self-Help Course is designed to give you the knowledge and skills you need to take a more active part in your arthritis care.
4. Being responsible for your arthritis includes
   a. Keeping informed about your status—asking questions
   b. Taking part in planning the treatment program—telling the health care team about your preferences and goals
   c. Trying out different treatments (under the guidance of your health care team) until you come up with the best treatment program for you
   d. Setting goals and working toward them
   e. Informing the health care team about problems and changes you make in your daily program

Activity 3: DEBUNKING MYTHS (10 min.)

Methods: Lecturette and quiz

1. As we pointed out in our preview of the course content, we will be learning and using different strategies to manage our arthritis. Before we begin exploring these, however, we would

like you to answer some questions which reflect some beliefs about arthritis.

2. Ask participants to write whether or not they agree, partially agree, or disagree with the following statements about arthritis. Tell them their answers will *not* be collected. Do not take more than a few minutes to complete this exercise. Read the following:

   a. If you are feeling tired or fatigued, you should always rest.

   b. If exercise hurts, you should not exercise.

   c. The best diet for someone with arthritis is one low in fats and high in fiber.

   d. One can easily injure joints by exercising.

   e. Arthritis pain is caused mainly by damaged joints.

   f. Health professionals are the best people to solve arthritis problems.

3. After the group has finished writing their responses, cover the following explanations. Note that these are based on what we now know from the latest arthritis research. Mention again that these topics will be discussed more completely in later sessions, referring to Chart 3. Responses:

   a. While fatigue is a symptom of the disease process, feeling tired can also be caused by stress or other emotions. Therefore, many people may find that exercise actually gives them more energy and that rest is not always appropriate.

   b. Many times people confuse arthritis pain with exercise-induced pain caused by weak or sore muscles. We will talk more about the difference between these in the next class and provide some guidelines for telling them apart. Exercising will actually help lessen the pain when done correctly, but if you allow the pain to stop you from ever starting, you will not get anywhere. The bottom line is that if you can move, you can exercise.

   c. A diet low in fats and high in fiber is desirable for good health in general. Diets recommended by the Heart Foundation and the Anti-Cancer Council are good ones to follow. There is no specific "arthritis" diet.

d. It is very difficult to cause permanent damage to joints by exercising. In fact, by using the proper exercise techniques, the joint is strengthened and supported better, not damaged. Exercises such as walking, swimming, and bicycling can all help arthritis and contribute to overall improved fitness.

e. Some arthritis pain is caused by damaged joints. However, much of arthritis pain is also caused by stress, tight or weak muscles, and emotions. In this course, we will learn ways to deal with all kinds of arthritis pain.

f. Only you can solve your problems. Health professionals, family, and friends can all make suggestions. However, only you make the final decisions about what to do and how to carry out your program. You are in charge!

BREAK (10 min.)

Activity 4: INTRODUCTION TO ARTHRITIS (15 min.)

Background Reading: *Helpbook,* pp. 1-16
Methods: Lecturette and discussion
Note: Refer to picture of joint on page 2 of *Helpbook*

1. Classic definition of *arthritis*—diseases of joints.
2. If anything goes wrong with any part of the joint, it is usually arthritis.
3. Now known to be not one disease but more than 100 different diseases.
4. No known cure for most forms of arthritis; therefore, self-management of symptoms is important.

5. Anatomy of joint: bone, muscle, cartilage, tendon, bursa, and synovial membrane (see *Helpbook,* p. 2).
6. Difference between osteoarthritis (OA) and rheumatoid arthritis (RA) (see table below). Have participants refer to page 3 of the *Helpbook.*

	Osteoarthritis	*Rheumatoid Arthritis*
Pathology: what happens	Cartilage degeneration; bone regeneration (spurs).	Inflammation of synovial membrane, bone destruction, damage to ligaments, tendons.
Joints affected	Hands, spine, knees, hips. May be asymmetrical (one-sided).	Wrists, knees, knuckles; symmetrical (both sides).
Features	Localized pain, stiffness, Heberdeen's nodules; usually not much swelling.	Swelling, redness, warmth, pain, tenderness, nodules, fatigue, stiffness, muscle aches, fever.
Prognosis	Less pain for some, more for others. Few severely disabled.	Less aggressive with time; deformity can often be prevented.
Age of onset	Age 45-90. Most of us have some features with increasing age.	Adults in 20s-50s.
Sex, heredity	Males and females equally. The form with knobby fingers runs in families.	75% female, 1/2 of 1% of U.S. population. Family tendency.
Tests	X-rays.	Rheumatoid factor (80%), blood tests, X-rays, examination of joint fluid.
Treatment	Maintain activity level, exercise, joint protection, relaxation, heat, sometimes medication and/or surgery.	Reduce inflammation, balanced exercise program, weight control, relaxation, heat, usually medication, sometimes surgery.

NOTE: This section is deliberately brief. Encourage participants to read the *Helpbook* this week and bring any questions they have to the next class.

Activity 5: EXERCISE FOR FUN AND FITNESS
—WHERE TO START (20 min.)

Background Reading: *Helpbook,* pp. 35-47
Methods: Lecturette and discussion
Note: Refer to Chart 4

1. In this course, we will talk about exercise for fun and fitness. Just because you have arthritis is no reason why you should not be fit and enjoy exercise.
2. Brainstorm: What does it mean to be fit? After the brainstorm, be sure that these five points are covered:
   a. Strong cardiovascular system—heart and blood vessels
   b. Good strength
   c. Good endurance/stamina
   d. Good flexibility
   e. Low percentage of body fat—proper weight
3. A good fitness program accomplishes all of the above and more. It has 3 parts (refer to Chart 4).
4. A warm-up routine usually consists of some flexibility/ strengthening exercises and a gradual increase in aerobic activity. When you are able to do 15 minutes of flexibility/

Chart 4
3 PARTS OF A FITNESS PROGRAM

WARM-UP (for muscle strength and flexibility; preparation for aerobic exercise)
AEROBIC EXERCISE (for cardiovascular fitness, endurance, and weight control)
COOL-DOWN (for body relaxation and to avoid sore muscles)

strengthening exercises, you are ready to move on to your
aerobic activity. Remember to cool down afterward with a
gradual decrease in activity and some more flexibility/
strengthening exercise.

5. There are as many fitness programs as there are people. One
example is a warm-up that includes slow walking, followed by
a few minutes of brisker walking and then a few more minutes
of slow walking again. If you are just beginning a program, start
by walking slowly for 3-5 minutes. Build up gradually until you
can walk 15 minutes. If you can already walk 15 minutes, start
by walking slowly for 5-10 minutes, and then walk briskly for
5-20 minutes, ending with a slow walk to cool down for 5-10
minutes. The basic principle is to start by doing whatever you can
do now, 3-4 times a week, and build up from there gradually.

6. During this course, we want each of you to chart your fitness
progress. There are very few of us who in some way could not
be more fit. For homework this week, ask everyone to think
about how they would like to improve their fitness and be ready
to report on this next week, as well as on what they can do now.

Activity 6: CONTRACTING (20 min.)

Background Reading: *Helpbook,* pp. 27-33
Methods: Lecturette and discussion
Note: Refer to Chart 5.

1. Over the years, we have found that the self-helpers who accomplish the most are the ones who set short-term goals. Therefore, in this class we will be asking each of you to make a
contract each week for something *you* want to accomplish. For
example, a contract might be "This week I'll walk 3 blocks
before lunch on 4 days," or "This week I will not eat after dinner
4 nights," or "This week I will practice relaxation techniques
for 15 minutes 3 nights after dinner."

Chart 5
RULES OF CONTRACTING

1. **IDENTIFY SOMETHING YOU WANT TO DO.**
2. **BE REALISTIC.**
3. **SPECIFY—WHAT, WHEN, HOW MANY, OR HOW MUCH.**
4. **WRITE IT DOWN.**
5. **CHECK IT DAILY.**

---

2. Discuss the rules for making a contract (refer to Chart 5).

3. Leaders give examples of the contracts they will do in the next week.

4. If the group is more than 10, break the class into two groups, with one leader in each group.

5. Introduce participants to the contract form in their *Helpbook* (p. 33). Ask participants to write a contract for the week.

6. Have participants read their contracts and tell how confident they are that they can accomplish them (100 is *very certain,* 0 is *not at all certain*). Emphasize that this number is *not* the percentage of the contract they believe they can complete, but how certain they are that they can complete the *whole* contract. If 100 or 90, suggest the contract may be too easy. If 70 or less, suggest the contract may be too hard. In either case, suggest that the participant adjust the contract. (To help people contract, see box on facing page.)

7. If someone is having trouble writing a clear contract (i.e., specific activity, times per day, days per week), ask other group members for suggestions *before* you help. Do not spend more than 3-4 minutes with any one person. If someone is having problems, work with him or her individually after class.

8. While participants are still in contracting groups, have them close their eyes, take 3 deep breaths, and think about them-

How to Help Someone Make a Contract

Step 1: Deciding What One Wants to Accomplish

Ask the person, "What will you do this week?" It is important that the activity come from the participant and *not* you. This activity does not have to be something covered in class—just something that the participants want to do to change behavior. Do not let anyone say, "I will try. . . ." Each person should say, "I will. . . ."

Step 2: Making a Plan

This is the difficult and most important part of contracting. Step 1 is worthless without Step 2. The plan should contain all of the following elements:

1. *Exactly what* is the participant going to do (e.g., how far will you walk, how will you eat less, what relaxation techniques will you practice)?
2. *How much* (e.g., walk around the block, 15 minutes, etc.)?
3. *When* will the participant do this? Again, this must be specific (e.g., before lunch, in the shower, when I come home from work).
4. *How often* will the activity be done? This is a bit tricky. Most participants tend to say, "Every day." In contracting, the most important thing is to succeed. Therefore, it is better to contract to do something 4 times a week and exceed the contract by actually doing it 5 times than to contract to do something every day and fail by doing it only 6 days. To ensure success, we usually encourage people to contract to do something 3 to 5 days a week. Remember that success and self-efficacy are as important as, or maybe even more important than, actually doing the behavior.

Step 3: Checking the Contract

Once the contract is complete, ask the participant, "Given a scale of 0-100, with 0 being *totally unsure* and

continued overleaf

100 being *totally certain,* how certain are you that you will [repeat the participant's contract verbatim]?"

If the answer is 70 or above, this is probably a realistic contract, and the participant should write it on his or her contract sheet.

If the answer is below 70, then the contract should be reassessed. Ask the participant, "What makes you uncertain? What problems do you foresee?" Then discuss the problems. Ask other participants to offer solutions. *You should offer solutions last.* Once the problem solving is completed, have the participant restate the contract and return to repeat Step 3, checking the contract.

Notes: This contracting process may seem cumbersome and time consuming. However, it does work and is well worth the effort. The first time you contract with a group, plan 2 to 3 minutes per person. Contracting is a learned skill. Your participant will soon be saying, "I will _____ 4 times this week before lunch and am 80% certain I can do this." Thus, after two or three contracting sessions, contracting should take less than a minute per participant.

selves successfully fulfilling their contracts. Read Script 1 (see facing page; when reading the script wait a few seconds every time you see the dots . . .) or, if time permits, use the "Visualization to Achieve Your Goals" exercise on the leader's tape.

9. Inform the participants that the class leaders will be calling them once during the coming week to support them in their contract.

Activity 7: CLOSING (5 min.)

1. Invite participants to review what was covered today for next week in the *Helpbook*:

Chapters 1-3, pp. 1-16

Chapter 6, pp. 27-33

Script 1

Close your eyes. . . . Now take 3 deep breaths: in through your nose and out through your mouth. . . . See yourself carrying out the activity in your contract. . . . (30-45 seconds of silence). . . . Think about how good you feel. . . . Take 3 more deep breaths and open your eyes.

---

2. Remind participants to keep track of their contracts daily and to bring them to class next week.

3. Remind participants to think about what they will do to gain greater fitness and be ready to report this next week.

4. Ask participants to bring their books to class each week. Also ask them to bring a tape measure or yardstick next week.

5. Tell people to wear comfortable clothes in which they can practice exercises, and ask if 2-4 people will bring blankets that can be put on the floor for exercise. Assure people that the exercise will not be strenuous and no one has to do anything they do not want to do.

6. Thank people for coming and tell them that one of the leaders will be calling them during the week to see how things are going.

7. Collect name tags.

8. Stay around for 15 minutes or so to answer questions and straighten the room.

¤ BIBLIOGRAPHY

Lorig, K., & Fries, J. (1995). *The arthritis helpbook* (5th ed.). Reading, MA: Addison-Wesley.

4

Selecting, Preparing, and Using Materials

Cecilia Doak
Leonard Doak
Kate Lorig

Patient education materials can stand alone or can be used to supplement other types of patient education. They can be as simple as directions on how to take a medication or as complex as surgical procedures. They have value only if the materials accomplish what they are produced to accomplish. Their value has little to do with sophistication, technology, or glitz.

Like all other aspects of patient education, materials must be produced on the basis of a needs assessment that results in specific objectives to be met by the materials (see Chapter 1). The value of educational materials is not judged by entertainment value or patient satisfaction. Rather, it is based on how well the materials meet their objectives (see Chapter 3).

When deciding to use materials, you must first decide whether you will use existing materials or create your own. Among the criteria for judging patient education material, three are especially important: (a) The material contains the information that the patient wants, (b) the material contains the information that the patient needs, and (c) the patient understands and uses the material as presented. Let us examine the application of these criteria.

¤ DOES THE MATERIAL CONTAIN THE INFORMATION THE PATIENT WANTS?

The only way to answer this question is by needs assessment before preparing or choosing material (see Chapter 1). Needs assessments may give you new insights into the appropriate use of material. For example, an assessment of people with asthma suggested that two problems often overlooked are anger and the stigma of having to use an inhaler in public. On the other hand, the needs assessment revealed that patients had little desire for more than very basic knowledge about how lungs function. Most asthma education materials do not address the problems of anger or the embarrassment caused by using an inhaler. They do, however, contain a great deal of information on pulmonary anatomy and physiology.

Another example was a needs assessment conducted with arthritis patients whose primary language was Spanish. They

TABLE 4.1 Health Care Professional Focus Versus Patient Focus

Health Care Professional Focus	Patient Focus
Anatomy and physiology (symptoms)	Why do I feel bad?
Necessary behaviors to maintain or improve health	Behaviors to solve problems caused by the disease
Facts about the disease	Beliefs about the disease
Skills necessary to carry out health-related behaviors	Skills necessary to maintain a "normal" life
Frustration that patients do not do what they should	Frustration/fear/depression about living with the disease
Fear about malpractice	Fear about the future

complained that it was very difficult for them to get good information about their disease. Materials written in English were not usable because of language. Health care providers did not speak Spanish or had very limited time. Finally, materials that were available in Spanish were simplified and brief. The Spanish-speaking patients wanted written materials that were clearly written, yet comprehensive. As a result of this assessment, the patient educators changed their plans from preparing a booklet in Spanish to writing a full-length book.

Needs assessments also provide us with information on how to frame our material. For example, we might use a question-and-answer format based on frequently asked patient questions or a problem-centered format based on patient problems. The importance of framing materials in the context of patient thinking rather than professional thinking cannot be overemphasized. A person recovering from a stroke will be more interested in "doing what you like" than in "your daily exercises."

Table 4.1 points out the different ways patients and health care professionals view the information contained in health materials. The material you prepare or choose should reflect the way patients think about health problems.

¤ DOES THE MATERIAL CONTAIN THE
INFORMATION THE PATIENT NEEDS?

This question is not easy to answer. Most professionals think that they know what patients need to know. In fact, we are so sure we "know" what is best that we seldom question our assumptions. This can lead to some serious problems. For example, a young man facing a hip replacement was taught how to use a walker and how to use a backpack to move his belongings. Neither of these skills, however, prepared him to move his soup from the stove to the table.

A basic skill needed by diabetics is glucose monitoring. Yet we know that many diabetics, even after all our best efforts, never monitor their glucose. In this case, the problem is not needing to know how to monitor glucose. We should also be teaching other skills that will help the diabetic and be more acceptable to the patient, such as how to balance medication, food, and exercise in such a way that life can be pleasurable despite the disease. Another emphasis may be on overcoming barriers to glucose monitoring. We must come to terms with the fact that some skills or information that the patient "needs to know" may not be acceptable to the patient. In this case, we might consider reworking the information so it is a better match for the tasks the patient has to carry out.

To decide what information the patient needs to know, use the first two steps in priority setting found in Chapter 3 (section "Setting Priorities"). We must be careful to ensure that the information is not too inclusive or exclusive. Sometimes, we put in too much and confuse the patient. In other cases, we do not supply all the information necessary to carry out the behaviors. For example, we usually tell patients when to take their medications, but we often forget to tell them what to do if they forget a dose or get off schedule. Instructions should include not only ideal circumstances but also real circumstances.

¤ CAN THE PATIENT UNDERSTAND THE MATERIAL AS PRESENTED?

The best way to answer this question is to ask patients. Use questions that reveal comprehension, such as "What does this material tell you about _____ (subject)? What does it tell you to do?" Do not ask, "Do you understand?" because a "yes" answer does not tell you *what* they understand. Patients often use "yes" as an easy way to avoid more questions.

Too often health professionals preempt patients and make decisions about what *they* think patients can or cannot understand. The most reliable way to find out if material is understandable is to have representative patients or groups of patients use the material and give feedback on *what* they understand. This can be done through structured interviews or focus groups (see Chapter 1).

When we were writing a book for Spanish-speaking arthritis patients, we were concerned that there would be too much material or that the material would be at a level that was not easily understandable. But when we tested the book with a group of patients, we found a very different problem. The patients wanted more than one picture of each exercise. One drawing was not always enough for them to understand what to do. No one was concerned with the 200 pages of written text, even though some people in the test group had only a year or two of schooling. These people told us that they wanted the information and that if they had a difficult time reading it, they would get help.

In short, there is no way around field testing. This is important whether you prepare your own material or choose materials that have been prepared by others. There is no shortage of patient education materials today. They are prepared by voluntary health associations such as the Cancer Society and the Lung Association. There are even materials for rarer conditions such as scleroderma and Gaucher disease. In addition, many commercial companies as well as drug companies publish patient education materials. The problem is choosing which ones are suitable for your patients. By applying the three criteria discussed, you will make this task easier.

One way to predict the ease or difficulty your patients may have with written material is to determine its literacy demand or its readability level. Is it likely to be too easy or over the heads of your intended audience? Readability formulas and the Suitability Assessment of Materials (Doak, Doak, & Root, 1995) are two means of determining this.

Readability Formulas

You can determine the reading level of your material by using a simple formula based on just two factors: the number of words in a sentence and the number of syllables in the words. These factors predict the level of literacy needed for reading the material. Other tests such as the Cloze readability formula (Spadero, Robinson, & Smith, 1980) tell how well adults understand specific patient education materials.

Why is it a good idea to test your material? Many health professionals write for patients as if they were writing for scientific journals. The application of a readability formula will help convince them that the material may not be understandable and needs to be revised. Most of all, a formula gives you an objective measure of the reading level of your material. You can then judge how this might affect your audience. For example, if you are aiming material at people with an average of 4 years of formal education, university-level material will turn them off very quickly. Don't worry that good readers will feel talked down to by instruction with a low reading level. Research and experience show that adults at all reading skill levels prefer, remember better with, and learn faster with easy-to-read instructions.

An attainable goal for most health care instructions is the sixth-grade level. About 75% of adult Americans will be able to follow instructions reasonably well at this level.

Nearly all of the 40-plus different readability formulas provide a reasonably accurate grade level (typically plus or minus one grade level with a 68% confidence factor). The authors recommend the Fry formula (Fry, 1968), which applies from Grade 1 through Grade 17 (university level) and does not require an extensive test sample of the material. Over a dozen computer programs are also available.

You do not have to test the readability of every word and sentence. Because reading levels vary considerably from one part of your material to another, select three samples from different content topics, if possible. Select text, not tables, figures, word lists, or graphics.

Figure 4.1 is a graph for estimating readability, along with directions for use.

Can the formulas in English be used for foreign languages? No; the sentence construction, number of words with many syllables, and so forth vary markedly in different languages. Zakaluk and Samuels (1988) have published formulas in 11 different languages, but some have not been validated with large samples. The original purpose of readability formulas was for use in the elementary classroom to guide placement of students in developing reading skills.

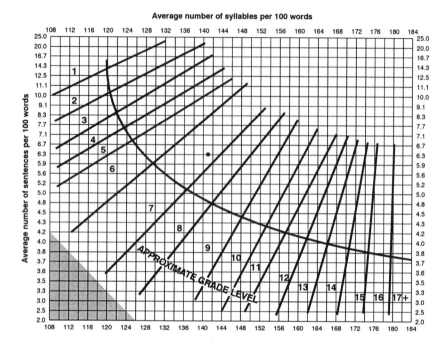

Average number of syllables per 100 words

Directions: Randomly select 3 one hundred word passages from a book or an article. Plot average number of syllables and average number of sentences per 100 words on graph to determine the grade level of the material. Choose more passages per book if great variablility is observed and conclude that the book has uneven readability. Few books will fall in gray area but when they do grade levels are invalid.

Count proper nouns, numerals, and initializations as words. Count a syllable for each symbol. For example, 1945 is 1 word and 4 syllables and IRA is 1 word and 3 syllables.

Example:	*Syllables*	*Sentences*
1st hundred words	124	66
2nd hundred words	141	55
3rd hundred words	158	68
Average	141	63

Readability: 7th Grade (see dot plotted on graph)

Figure 4.1. Fry Graph for Estimating Readability—Extended

SOURCE: "Fry's Readability Graph: Clarification, Validity, and Extension to Level 17," by E. Fry, 1977, *Journal of Reading, 11*, pp. 242-252. Copyright 1977 by the International Reading Association. Reprinted by permission.

The Suitability Assessment of Materials

Understanding depends upon more than the words and sentences. If the material looks hard to read or has too many facts jammed into a paragraph, it may be cast aside without another glance. To help you take into account the variety of factors that influence people in understanding material, we provide below a condensed version of a list called the Suitability Assessment of Materials (SAM; Doak et al., 1995).

The list is divided into six sections: content, literacy demand, graphics, layout and typography, learning stimulation and motivation, and cultural appropriateness. Each section has criteria to be applied to your material.

1. Content
   a. Can patients easily understand the intended *purpose* of the material? If they cannot, they may not pay attention, or they may miss the main point.
   b. Is there clear, behavior-specific *content* that helps patients solve their problems? (For more discussion, see earlier sections of this chapter.)
   c. Is the *scope* limited to the objectives? One problem with many materials is that they contain more information than patients need, want, or can reasonably learn.
   d. Is there a *review* or *summary* of the key points? This is important, as readers often miss the key points on first exposure.
2. Literacy demands
   a. Is the material written at an *appropriate readability level?* (see the discussion of readability formulas earlier in this chapter).
   b. Is the material presented in a *conversational style using the active voice?* Long or multiple phrases included in a sentence slow down the reading process and generally make comprehension more difficult.

   c. Does the material use *common and explicit words?* For example:

- *doctor* rather than *physician*
- *use* rather than *utilize*
- *heart disease* rather than *coronary artery disease*
- *beans* rather than *legumes*
- *15-70* rather than *normal range*
- *pain lasting more than 5 minutes* rather than *excessive pain*

Whenever possible, use image words or analogies. These are things people can "see" or "feel." For example, *vegetables* is better than *dietary fiber,* and *a runny nose* is better than *excessive mucus.*

   d. Is the *context* given before new information? We learn new facts/behaviors more quickly when told the context first: for example, "To find out what is wrong with you [the context first], the technician will take a sample of your blood for lab tests [new information]."

   e. Are there *advance organizers* (road signs)? Headers or topic captions tell briefly what is coming up next. These advance organizers make material look less formidable and also prepare one's thought process to expect the next topic. They also help busy readers pick and choose what they want to read.

  3. Graphics (illustrations, lists, tables, charts, graphs)

   a. Is the *cover graphic engaging?* Does it *convey* the message you want to convey? People do judge a booklet by its cover. This is a place to be especially careful. Does the cover graphic show what the material is all about?

   b. Are the *illustrations simple, realistic, and without distracting details?* Visuals are accepted and remembered better when they portray the familiar. Viewers may not recognize the meaning of medieval textbook drawings or abstract art/symbols. Photos should be limited in the amount of detail shown. Nonessential details such as room background, elaborate borders, and unnecessary color can be distracting.

   c. Do the illustrations tell the *key points* visually?

   d. Are all *graphics* (lists, tables, graphs, charts, geometric forms) *carefully and fully explained* in text near the graphic? Explanation and directions are essential and do little good if they are not in close proximity to the graphic.

   e. *Are captions used* to announce/explain graphics and illustrations? Captions can quickly tell the reader what the graphic or illustration is all about. A graphic without a caption is usually an inferior instruction and represents a missed learning opportunity.

4. Layout and typography

   a. *Are illustrations near related text?*

   b. Are there *usual cueing devices* such as boxes or arrows to point to the key information?

   c. Is there *adequate white space?*

   d. Does the material *look cluttered?*

   e. Is there *high contrast* between the ink and the paper? (This is especially important for older people and those with visual problems.)

   f. Are more than six type fonts or sizes used on one page? Too many fonts and sizes make the material appear confusing.

   g. Are all CAPS used? Type in all caps slows down reading comprehension for readers at all skill levels.

   h. Are there more than five to seven subheadings? Few people can remember more than seven independent items. For adults with lower literacy skills, the limit may be three to five items. Longer lists need to be partitioned into smaller "chunks."

5. Learning stimulation motivation

    a. *Is interaction included in the text and/or graphic?* Readers/viewers should be asked to *do something* (solve problems, make choices, demonstrate, etc.).

    b. Are desired *behaviors shown in specific terms* and modeled? People learn more readily by observation and doing rather than by reading or being told.

    c. *Are the behaviors presented as doable?* People are more motivated when they believe the tasks are doable. Telling people with emphysema to "exercise" is not very motivating. Telling them that "everyone can walk 10 minutes a day by walking 1 minute for each hour that he or she is awake" is much more motivating.

6. Cultural appropriateness

    a. Do the language, logic, experience, and illustrations *match* the language, logic, and experience of the population?

    b. *Are the cultural images positive, realistic, and appropriate?* Using Grandma Moses as an example of successful aging may be meaningless to a Hispanic population.

    c. *Does the material convey respect?* There is a tendency to infantilize materials for people from other cultures. People with low literacy or those who speak another language have the same ability to learn if taught appropriately.

The above list was developed to evaluate materials that are already written. It can also be used as a guide when preparing new materials. A word of caution, however: This is not a template for preparing materials. Rather, it is a guide. Read it over, prepare your materials, and then check them out to see if you have missed anything important.

¤ SUMMARY

Written material can be a very important patient education tool. However, like all patient education, it must be prepared and used with care and thought. This chapter should start you on your way.

¤ BIBLIOGRAPHY

Doak, C., Doak, L., & Root, J. H. (1995). *Teaching patients with low literacy skills* (2nd ed.). Philadelphia: J. B. Lippincott.

Fry, E. (1968). A readability formula that saves time. *Journal of Reading, 2,* 513-516, 575-578.

Gopen, G. D., & Swan, J. A. (1990). The science of scientific writing. *American Scientist, 78,* 550-558.

Miller, G. A. (1956). The magical number seven, plus or minus two: Some limits on our capacity for processing information. *Psychological Review, 63,* 81-87.

Spadero, D. C., Robinson, L. A., & Smith, L. A. (1980). Assessing readability of patient education materials. *American Journal of Hospital Pharmacy, 37,* 215-221.

White, J. V. (1988). *Graphic design for the electronic age: The manual for traditional and desktop publishing.* New York: Watson-Guptil.

Zakaluk, B. L., & Samuels, S. J. (1988). *Readability: Its past, present, and future.* Newark, DE: International Reading Association.

5

How Do I Get
People to Come?

Virginia M. González
Kate Lorig

The best patient education program in the world does no one any good if no one comes. Low attendance can occur for many reasons. You may have created a product no one wants, people may not know about your program, there may be factors that inhibit people from coming, or people may be actively discouraged from attending. In this chapter, we examine ways of marketing your program to health professionals, patients, and special populations that are hard to reach. Finally, we discuss some ways to use community resources to enhance your programs.

¤ MARKETING TO HEALTH PROFESSIONALS

Probably the strongest potential allies in marketing your program are other health professionals. At best, they can be very helpful. To be successful, you want to be sure that they are, at least, neutral. At worst, other professionals can completely destroy the program. With this in mind, let us start by examining how to get support from doctors and other health professionals. The time to start your marketing is when you plan your program. In Chapter 1, we talked about an interested-parties analysis; this is a good technique to involve health professionals.

With health professionals, it is important not only to get their input but also to let them be partners in the creation of your program. This does not mean endless group meetings. Rather, when you write content that would be of interest to a doctor, a physical therapist, or a nurse, have two or three key health professionals review it. Have a physician, a nurse, and a physical therapist review the whole program, offer comments, and suggest changes. In choosing your reviewers, do not just choose your friends. Rather, look for opinion leaders, health professionals who are highly respected by their peers. These might be instructors in health professional programs, officers in professional organizations, or senior, well-liked doctors. If your community has factions—for example, two hospitals— then choose reviewers from each faction.

Not only do you want health professionals as reviewers, but you also want to give these people ownership of the program. Ask if you can use their names on handouts or in publicity. When you write to other health professionals about the program, see if your reviewers will co-sign your letter. A program invented by Howard Doe, Helen Doe, M.D., Chief of Medicine, and Robin Doe, Head PT, may be easily introduced, as it comes from credible sources.

Anyone who has ever invented anything has come across the dreaded NIH syndrome, or Not Invented Here syndrome. You will recognize the symptoms when you hear "That may be the way they do it in New Zealand but not here in Australia," "Those people in California just do not understand our health system," or "People here are different." The quickest way to defuse this situation is to ask the "locals" to review the program and work with them to make any specific local adaptations. This forces the locals to look carefully at the program, rather than disliking it from afar. The revisions they make are usually very minor and may even help market the program locally. Most important of all, the local professionals now have ownership of the course, so NIH becomes IH—that is, Invented Here.

A second problem we often hear about is "We can not get doctors and other health professionals to refer people to our programs." If you survive the NIH syndrome, then the problem is probably that your professionals forget, find making a referral too complicated, or just do not have the time. Today, most health professionals are very busy. They have very little time and must prioritize what they tell patients. Most do not have adequate time to provide a diagnosis and treatment. Therefore patient education is not in the front of their minds. You may not be able to change this, but there are a couple of tricks you might try.

Place a poster about your program in the doctor's waiting room or examining room. Have patients tear off tags with the phone number for more information. This way, the doctor does not have to do anything, yet the patient understands that the doctor approves of the program. In addition, the poster acts as a stimulus for the patient to ask the doctor for more information or reminds the doctor about the program. Be sure to institute a system to replace these posters regularly.

A second method of enlisting help with recruitment from doctors and other health professionals is to place a brightly colored sign-up sheet in the waiting room. The front of the sheet should say something like "I am interested in learning more about diabetes education," with spaces for name, address, and phone number. The other side of the sheet is preaddressed and prestamped. Every 2 weeks, or when the sheet is full, whichever occurs first, the office receptionist takes down the sheet and mails it to you. In turn, he or she gets a new sheet. This takes all the responsibility away from the doctor and gets you the information you need. By the way, thank-you notes and an occasional small gift go a long way toward getting the cooperation of overworked and often underappreciated office staff.

A third method of getting doctor referrals is to make up special prescription pads (small printers can do this inexpensively). The doctor then prescribes patient education in much the same way he or she would prescribe medication. Some programs require a doctor's signature before people can attend. If this is the case, include a place on the physician referral (permission) form where the doctor can request material about the program for his or her office (see Figure 5.1).

Finally, some health plans, hospitals, or clinics have a newsletter in which you can advertise your program. Because it comes from a respected source, your program is also acceptable. When using a newsletter, be very sure your telephone number is published. Telling people about your program does no good if they do not know how to contact you.

Sometimes doctors fear that the education program will somehow interfere with their treatment or chase patients into the hands of another practitioner. To overcome this fear, first assure the doctors that you will always refer their patients back

Self-Management Study

Stanford University School of Medicine
Department of Medicine

Please return to:

Stanford Patient Education Research Center
1000 Welch Road, Suite 204
Palo Alto, California 94304
(415) 723-7935
(415) 723-9656 FAX

Patient's Name: _____

Address: _____

DIAGNOSIS: My patient has one or more of the following diseases and is age 40 or over. He/she does not have compromised mentation nor has he/she received radiation or chemotherapy for cancer within the past year.

PLEASE CHECK ALL DIAGNOSES THAT APPLY:

☐ Asthma

☐ Chronic bronchitis

☐ Emphysema/COPD

☐ Other chronic lung disease

    *Specify type:*_____

☐ Coronary artery disease

    with angina or congestive

    heart failure

☐ Completed cerebrovascular accident **with** neurological handicap and normal mentation

☐ Osteoarthritis

☐ Rheumatoid arthritis

☐ Other rheumatic disease

    *Specify type:*_____

☐ Other chronic disease

    *Specify type:*_____

_____   _____
    DATE   SIGNATURE OF PHYSICIAN

                _____
                    PRINT name of physician

I am interested in referring patients to your study. Please send me:
  ☐ **Brochures**   #_____
  ☐ **Exam room posters** #_____
  ☐ **Prescription pads** #_____
My address is:

Figure 5.1. Sample Physician Referral Form for a Patient Education Program

to them. And be sure to do so. Second, you might offer to hold the program after hours in the doctor's waiting room. This solves your space problem and ensures that a specific doctor is associated with that session of the program.

These days, patient data are often computerized. This is especially true under managed care. Sometimes you can sort these data to target the patients you want and mail a letter directly to them. Of course, care must be taken to maintain confidentiality. It is best if the letters can come from the physician, clinic, or health plan. (Figure 5.2 shows a sample letter.)

Within your program, and in your dealings with the public, be very sure to teach that the doctor is not the enemy. Too often, there is a subtle or not-so-subtle implication that the patient must be on the defensive with doctors. Avoid this at all costs. Also, do not play favorites. Even though you may like one doctor better than another, *always* support the patient's choice of doctor. If there are medical questions, suggest that the patient ask his or her doctor. If a patient is unhappy with the doctor, urge a patient-doctor discussion. A doctor once said that doctors will get off their pedestals when patients get off their knees. Our job is to help patients stand, not to knock doctors off their pedestals.

¤ MARKETING TO THE PUBLIC

Making Your Program Attractive

Much of the problem in recruiting patients is that your program is not attractive. Some of the common problems are the program's name, cost, time, place, and length.

Stanford Patient Education Research Center

Stanford University School of Medicine
Department of Medicine

1000 Welch Road, Suite 204
Palo Alto, California 94304
(415) 723-7935
(415) 723-9656 FAX

March 20, 1995

Dear Patient:

Your Stanford Health Service Pulmonary Disease Clinic is supporting an educational program being conducted by our Stanford Patient Education Research Center. We are writing to encourage you to participate in the Self-Management Course for people with heart conditions, lung conditions, arthritis or stroke. A brief description of the Self-Management Course is enclosed.

Many previous course participants with lung disease have experienced less limitation in activity and physical capability, have had less depression and distress about their disease, and have had less dependence upon physicians. Quite possibly, you would experience the same benefits.

Participation will not interfere in any way with your current treatment or with your relationship with your physician. Any benefits you may receive from participation will be in addition to those you are receiving from your current treatment.

There will be no cost to you for participating. Courses are held in locations near your home.

If you are interested in participating, please return the enclosed postcard. If you have questions, call the Patient Education Center at 1-800-DO-MANAGE (1-800-366-2624).

Sincerely,

Halsted Holman, M.D
Professor of Medicine

Kate Lorig, R.N., Dr.P.H.
Project Director

Figure 5.2. Sample Letter to Patients About a Patient Education Program

Name

The title of your program is very important. "Self-Help for the Elderly" forces participants to admit they are old before enrolling. "Growing Younger and Healthier" might be a better title. Hypertension is a symptomless disease, so there may be little motivation on the part of many patients to attend a program. On the other hand, chronic obstructive pulmonary disease (COPD) has painful symptoms; therefore it might be easier to recruit for "COPD Better Breathers" programs. Sometimes programs with more than one focus can help. Because a large percentage of older people have arthritis, you might reach more elderly hypertensives with an arthritis/high blood pressure program than with just a high blood pressure program. One way to choose a name while also resolving some of the other issues discussed in this section is by using focus groups. You will find details about these in Chapter 1.

Some final hints about naming programs:

- Do not be too "cute." Illness is a serious matter, especially to the ill. Treating it frivolously often causes anger.
- Keep the name simple. No one wants to deal with a 14-word name.
- Make the name descriptive. The name is what initially attracts people. "Asthma Self-Management," "Avoiding Heart Attacks," "How to Talk With Your Doctor," and "Preparing for Labor" are all good, clear, descriptive titles. "Aches and Pains" is cute, but not very descriptive.

Cost

There is a widely held belief among health professionals and others that if people pay for something, they value it more.

Although this may be true, we have little evidence to suggest that payment makes much difference in terms of behavior change or health status outcome. In fact, if payment were directly linked to outcome, the United States would have the healthiest population in the world! The point here is that you do not have to charge money to make patients appreciate your program. On the other hand, payment may influence attendance or commitment. For example, some weight loss programs charge a high fee and then offer rebates for prespecified weight loss and weight loss maintenance.

You may need to charge to cover the expenses of the program. Usually, the lower or more minimal the fee, the better. This makes your program accessible to everyone. If you must charge more than a minimal fee, you might try a sliding scale. Your application can state that the program costs $25 but that considerations will be made for those with a limited income. Then, as part of the application, have participants check one of the following:

Enclosed is $25.00.
I can afford only $___; enclosed is $___.
Please consider me for a fee waiver ___.

If the fee is reasonable, the public does not take advantage of this offer. In my experience with an arthritis patient education program (the Arthritis Self-Help Course), most people pay the full fee and very few request a complete scholarship. When we have charged $15 to $20, fewer than 5% of over 1,000 patients have asked for a fee waiver. All the rest have paid the full fee. When the cost of the course is raised to $30 to $40, attendance is badly affected. Today, with the spread of HMOs and other prepaid plans, patient education is often budgeted as part of ongoing patient services. If this is not true in your area, part of your job is advocating for formal patient education to be a part of ongoing budgeted services. Often some of the course expenses can be paid for from other sources. For more information, see the section "Using Community Resources" later in this chapter.

Time

It seems obvious that you should hold your program at a convenient time for the clients. Saturday may be a sports day for you but a very lonely day for the elderly. Also, take a look at your competition. Do not hold your hypertension program during the Olympics or on a church bingo night. However, it might be successful to hold it at the bingo hall a half hour before bingo. You may even consider offering more than one program on different days, at different times, in order to reach more people.

You should also consider the length of your program. Once programs get to be longer than 5 to 7 weeks, completion is a problem. Although 2 hours a week for 5 or 6 weeks may be convenient for city dwellers, people in rural areas who must travel a distance may find it more convenient to attend two half-day sessions.

Place

People are funny. Some places are all right to go to and others are not. This has nothing to do with safety. If you want to reach an ethnic population, you might have more success holding the program in a community setting rather than the hospital. Some Catholics may not go to a Protestant church for a program or vice versa, and others will. Also, some people may cross town for a program but not cross the railroad tracks. People have a range, and your program must be given within the range of your audience. Your task is to find out what that range is, perhaps through your needs assessment or in a focus group.

Of course, sites must be safe and accessible. Things to consider are stairs, impediments to the physically challenged, parking, public transportation, walking distance, lighting, comfort of chairs, accessibility of toilets, and facilities for making coffee and tea. If you are teaching wellness or prevention, hospitals may not be the best places because, in people's minds, that is where sick people go. Hospitals have a negative image for some people. They are also full of "strange, frightening things" and peculiar smells. In addition, parking and access for the general pubic may require a lot of walking. For this reason, try to hold your course on neutral ground. Shopping malls, pubs, hotels, town halls, senior centers, and libraries usually meet this criterion. They are accessible and acceptable to a wide spectrum of the population (see the section "Using Community Resources" later in this chapter).

Using the Media

So you have done everything right, and still no one comes. It may be that no one knew about your program. Good advertising is done in a number of ways. The local media, radio and newspapers, are excellent but also unpredictable if you rely solely on public service announcements. The problem is that you never know when your announcement will get published or be announced. Nevertheless, you should send press releases to all your local media. These should be short and ready to use. See Figures 5.3 and 5.4 for some examples of press releases. Unfortunately, paid advertising is very expensive. However, for

Self-Management Study

Stanford University School of Medicine
Department of Medicine

Stanford Patient Education Research Center
1000 Welch Road, Suite 204
Palo Alto, California 94304
(415) 723-7935
(415) 723-9656 FAX

PRESS RELEASE
PSA

March, 1995

Contact: Kate Lorig, RN, Dr P.H.
             (415) 723-7935

****

SELF-MANAGEMENT PROGRAM

FOR HEART CONDITIONS, LUNG CONDITIONS, ARTHRITIS, STROKE

Fatigue, frustration, pain, limitations? If so, this Self-Management Course has been designed just for you. The course, developed by the Stanford University School of Medicine's Patient Education Research Center, teaches people 40 and over to cope with the symptoms and frustrations of living with a chronic condition. The course is offered four times a year at various locations in San Francisco, San Mateo, Santa Clara and Alameda counties. The next session of classes begins in April. There is no charge. Enrollment is limited and pre-registration is required. For more information, contact the Stanford Patient Education Research Center at **1-800 DO MANAGE or 1-800-366-2624.##**

Figure 5.3. Sample Press Release on a Patient Education Program

SLANFORD ARTHRITIS CENTER   STANFORD UNIVERSITY SCHOOL OF MEDICINE   Department of Medicine

PRESS RELEASE
PSA

February, 1995

Contact: Steven L. Wilson
             Program Coordinator
             (415) 723-7935

ARTHRITIS SELF-MANAGEMENT

An internationally renowned arthritis course is now available to you. Over 200,000 people have enjoyed the benefits of the Arthritis Self-Help Course, sponsored by the Arthritis Foundation. This is a six week course offered twice each year at various locations in San Francisco, San Mateo, Santa Clara, San Benito, Santa Cruz and Monterey counties.

In the course you will learn about arthritis, its medications and the latest in exercise and pain management techniques for people with arthritis. You will learn how to work effectively with your physician. You will also design and carry out your own self-management program while sharing your experiences with others. The next series begins this month. Pre-registration is required and enrollment is limited. The materials fee is $15.00 and fee waivers are available. Anyone with arthritis or other rheumatic diseases, their spouses or friends are welcome. If you would like more information call the Arthritis Foundation toll free at **1-800-283-7800**.##

ARTHRITIS SELF-HELP PROGRAM • STUDY ASSESSING THE PERSONAL IMPORTANCE TO PATIENTS OF CHANGES IN HEALTH STATUS • SPANISH ARTHRITIS SELF-MANAGEMENT STUDY

STANFORD ARTHRITIS CENTER · 1000 WELCH ROAD, SUITE 204 · PALO ALTO, CALIFORNIA 94304 · (415) 723-7935 · FAX (415) 723-9656

Figure 5.4. Sample Press Release on a Patient Education Program

something really important, this may be the way to go. Again, it is important to know the audience. You would not want to advertise a prenatal program for teens on an all-news radio station.

Sometimes when you are starting a new program or have a new angle on an old program, you can get the newspapers to do a feature story. If this happens, be sure that the story includes how you can be reached. The best story in the world is useless if your address or phone number is not included. On radio, the equivalent of a feature story is a short interview or, better still, a talk show. Again, it is important that you somehow get in the information on how to contact you. In fact, on radio, this should be done several times, as listeners may not get all the information the first time it is given.

Besides the large mass media, all communities have a number of club, church, and other newsletters. Putting your announcement in those targeted to your audience can be both effective and inexpensive. The problem with these is that they usually have a long lead time. Thus, if you want something published the first of January, it may have to be in by early November. Sometimes correspondence sent by fax receives more attention than that sent by mail. It is useful to keep a file of all media sources, contact persons, and lead times.

Flyers can also be effective if well placed. I have found that good places for flyers are on the cash registers at local pharmacies, in doctors' waiting rooms, at public libraries, in beauty and barber shops, and in local markets and shops. Sometimes, as in the case of an AIDS education program, it is helpful to hand out flyers on the street. Flyers can also be distributed by such organizations as Meals on Wheels. Sometimes you have to be really creative. If you are trying to reach a young audience, try putting flyers in fitness centers. Families with young children are often found in toy stores and fast food restaurants—advertise here. If you are trying to reach older populations, you might include a flyer in the program of the Sunday afternoon armchair travel program.

One final and excellent source of publicity is word of mouth. To use this, let past participants know about future programs. Ask them to post flyers in places that they frequent and also to tell their friends. You might even send people postcards that their friends can send in for more information. We have found this to be one of the very best sources of publicity.

Once you have gone through all the trouble of publicizing in many places, it is nice to know what is effective. The easiest way of doing this is having a place on your application for people to write in where they found out about your program. In this way, you can track your publicity and keep using those sources that are effective, while eliminating those that are not. Also be sure to ask anyone calling for information how he or she found out about your program.

Reaching the Hard to Reach

One of the biggest problems for many patient educators is reaching patients who are hard to reach. Often we consider those people who are not like ourselves or like our regular clients as being hard to reach. In English-speaking countries, most health care professionals speak English as their primary language; therefore the hard to reach might be defined as those whose primary language is not English. The poor and elderly are other groups that are defined as hard to reach.

In trying to identify ways to reach these groups, a good place to start is by looking at who is reaching them. Where and to whom do they go for information and service? By this we mean, where do they buy their food and clothing, and where are their social and sports activities? Why are these services successful when yours are not? At the same time, examine what happens when the "hard to reach" enter your health care system. Are there people who speak their language and understand their customs? Are your services located in a convenient place? Are people treated courteously? The ultimate question to ask yourself is "If I were them, would I use our services?"

In planning your program, you also want to ask yourself if you really want to reach them. This sounds harsh, but it is important to consider *before* beginning your outreach efforts. Really wanting to reach them means being willing and able to commit the resources—the staff, time, and money—to develop and maintain services in those communities. If you do not make efforts to provide ongoing funding or you pull out of a community too fast without helping that community develop resources and maintain the program, bad feelings, tension, and distrust are likely to result. This makes it difficult for anyone in the future to work in that community. Therefore establishing and maintaining good community relations are also important.

The primary rule in trying to reach the "hard to reach" is to go to them. Do not expect them to come to you. For more information on working competently with diverse cultures, see Chapter 6.

¤ USING COMMUNITY RESOURCES

Every community has resources. Finding them is the problem. Sometimes the problem is not really finding them but rather seeing what is before your eyes. For example, every community has hotels, bars, and restaurants. However, we seldom think of these as sites for patient education. In fact, many of these establishments spend a great deal of their time nearly empty. Thus you might be able to use a bar or a restaurant for a morning class. These sites might be especially attractive if you are trying to reach men. Hotel swimming pools are used heavily in the early morning and in the evenings. However, in between times, they might be used for a water exercise class. Similarly, doctors all have empty waiting rooms when patients are not being seen; these might be used for evening classes.

Service clubs are also common in most communities. Lions, Rotary, and Apex are all groups that can be called upon for help. One of the missions of these groups is community service. With a little creative thinking, you can help them fulfill their mission. Members of these organizations can be recruited to get people to courses or to give public lectures. Also, most communities have a variety of youth groups, such as Scouts and Guides. Members of these organizations can be trained as peer counselors or as babysitters for handicapped children or adults. They are also experts at distributing flyers or announcements. As a special project, they might even design some of your patient education materials. Give them a chance to do their daily good turn. Organizations such as police, firemen, unions, or farm clubs can also be most helpful.

In large communities, it is often difficult to get access to the media. However, just the opposite is sometimes true in smaller towns. Newspapers and radio stations need material. You may arrange to do a weekly newspaper column or a stress management program twice weekly over the radio. You will never find out what you can get if you do not ask.

Most merchants are constantly asked for things. Try asking for something different. For example, in a big city, ask a major department store to help you advertise an event. In turn, you can go through the store and help them identify products that they can feature for pregnant women, the elderly, the handicapped, and so on. Thus you are helping them to increase their customer base.

In places that are very hot, cold, or wet, walking and other outdoor exercises are sometimes a problem. Most of these same communities also have enclosed areas, be they malls, office buildings, airports, or markets. Such places can be used for walking programs in the hours before opening. In large cities, airports have miles of climate-controlled corridors that are good for walking. One elderly group walks inside a shopping mall two mornings a week from 8:00 to 9:00 and then has coffee and a health lecture in the mall coffee shop. Because there are few people in the mall as the shops open at 9:00, the owner is pleased to get the extra business. Walking tracks can be marked out with colored tape: Once around the mall equals a quarter mile, or two flights of stairs equals a 100-foot elevation gain.

You can find skilled personnel in much the same way as you find sites for your program. Many communities have volunteer bureaus. If you have special needs, ask. Many people would volunteer if they did not have to lick envelopes or be president of something. If there are no volunteer bureaus, make your needs known through church bulletins or the local newspaper. You never know what will happen.

All the above is fine and good, but what if what you really need is money? The place to start is near home. It is important to make clear to your organization that patient education is not merely a nice add-on service. It is an integral part of patient care. As such, it must be budgeted for in much the same way as nursing services. Good basic patient education programs usually cost one quarter to one half of 1% of an organization's total budget. This basic budget can be supplemented by service clubs, churches, grants from foundations, and merchants. Most of these organizations have planned giving programs, so they will not instantly hand over cash. However, if you understand their programs and how to ask for money through their channels, you may well get what you need.

Beyond local organizations, look to governmental groups: local, state, or national. Again, there are all kinds of rules and regulations. However, if you are willing to play the game and have a good product, you may well get the funding you need. In dealing with bureaucracies, remember to play by the rules: Dot all the i's and cross all the t's. Be sure that the government officials who will fund your request understand your program and are sold on it. After all, they will be the ones to present it to the people higher up. Finally, have enough time. You probably cannot find the funds you need in a week. However, any program that is worth doing today is probably also worth doing in 6 months.

No matter what you are asking for, one of the best ways to get it is by asking the person or organization you are approaching how to get what you want, the principle being that people usually want to be helpful. For example, if you want the local radio station to air a stress management series, ask the manager what you would need to do to get such a series on the air. He or she will then outline a number of things for you to do. Listen carefully and write these down. Then do just what he or she says. If you do this, it will be very difficult for him or her to keep the series off the air. When people tell you how to do something and you follow through, they have almost committed themselves to do it.

In short, all communities have resources. Your job is to recognize, find, and, most important, use them effectively.

¤ BIBLIOGRAPHY

"How-to" guides on community health promotion can be obtained from the Stanford Health Promotion Resource Center, 1000 Welch Road, Palo Alto, CA 94304. The following guides are available for $3.00 each or $54.75 for a set of 23 guides:

- Volunteers   No. HTP1
- Focus Groups   No. HTP2
- Placing Newspaper Ads   No. HTP3
- Writing and Sending Press Releases   No. HTP4
- Gaining Access to Media Resources   No. HTP5
- Working With Media Gatekeepers   No. HTP6
- Print Production: Dealing With Vendors   No. HTP7
- Building a Media Resources Inventory   No. HTP8
- Online Data Retrieval of Health Information   No. HTP9
- Conducting a Community Resource Inventory   No. HTP10
- Writing Effective Survey Questions   No. HTP11
- Building and Maintaining Effective Coalitions   No. HTP12
- Holding Press Conferences   No. HTP13
- Teambuilding for Community Health
  Promotion   No. HTP14
- Running Effective Meetings   No. HTP15
- Presenting Your Health Promotion Program   No. HTP16
- Institutionalization: Giving Programs a
  Permanent Base   No. HTP17
- Organizing Health Information   No. HTP18
- Writing up Your Program for Use by Others   No. HTP19
- How to Hire and Use a Consultant   No. HTP20
- Developing and Producing Brochures   No. HTP21
- Finding the Information You Need   No. HTP22
- Preparing for Media Interviews   No. HTP23

Working Cross-Culturally

Virginia M. González
Kate Lorig

Working cross-culturally can be challenging to even the most experienced health professional; it can also be some of the most interesting and rewarding work you will ever do. The way you approach the challenge will determine the success of your efforts. For example, if you choose to develop an educational program that respects and incorporates the cultural beliefs and practices of a group, you are more likely to be successful than if you simply translate or transplant an existing program from one group to another without making any adaptations.

In this chapter, we discuss some practical guidelines to help you work more effectively and comfortably with diverse cultural groups and to develop culturally appropriate patient education programs. Before we do that, however, it is important to explain what is meant by key concepts such as *culture, cultural identity,* and *ethnic identity* and how these contribute to diversity.

¤ UNDERSTANDING CULTURAL DIVERSITY

Culture is a shared set of beliefs, assumptions, values, and practices; it determines how we interpret and interact with the world and structures our behavior and attitudes throughout our lives. An individual's or group's culture strongly determines the way in which the individual or group defines health and illness. For example, in some cultural groups, health and illness are defined by the balance or imbalance of spiritual or supernatural forces rather than by biological, behavioral, or environmental factors alone. An appreciation and respect for these different beliefs and practices, as well as an understanding of how they differ from your own, will greatly enhance your ability to work with different cultural groups. This, in turn, will increase the effectiveness of your programs.

In planning and implementing patient education programs, it is important to realize that the individuals or groups you are targeting may actually have more than one cultural identity. Such variation in cultural identities within groups reflects the influence of several factors and individuals' responses to their experience with these factors:

• Historical, socioeconomic, and political experiences in the homeland and new country
• Education

- Family and peer influence
- Native or primary language
- Religion
- Age at time of immigration
- Place of residence and length of time in the new country
- Citizenship status
- Whether the individual lives in an integrated community

A person's cultural identity is dynamic, changing as a result of contact with different groups. This process of change, or acculturation, occurs naturally over time. It refers to the acquisition of a new cultural identity, but does not preclude retention of the old; a person may become bicultural, identifying with two different cultures (the old and new). Each individual has his or her own process of integrating the new culture with the old. Cultural diversity is the result of this interaction between different cultures. Individuals and groups create new cultural identities that are often a synthesis of separate and disparate cultures. For example, many immigrant groups have chosen to maintain the practices of their cultural heritage (i.e., their language, religion, and traditions) while also acquiring, to varying degrees and in different ways, some of the values, practices, and language of the new culture in order to function in the larger society.

The extreme form of acculturation is assimilation, in which the individual or group completely incorporates the new culture. Gradually, the values, practices, or traditions of the native culture, particularly those that do not conform to the standards of the new group, are lost or given up and replaced by those of the new group.

Understanding that diversity exists within and between cultures will help you avoid the tendency to form cultural stereotypes about a group with which you have had limited experience. One of the biggest mistakes you can make as a patient educator is to base your actions on inaccurate assumptions, misconceptions, oversimplifications, or generalizations about a patient's culture. By doing so, you might create a program or act in a way that is at best inappropriate and at worst offensive to the people you are trying to serve.

With this in mind, let's look at how to learn more about the cultural diversity of your patient population.

¤ WHERE TO START

If you are not sure which cultural groups you want to serve, start by gathering some specific information about your general patient population. For example, what are the demographic characteristics of the population? This includes information about age, sex, education, marital status, place of birth, ethnic origin, language spoken, type of health problems, and services used. Answers to these questions can help you better define your target groups, as well as learn something about their cultural identities and levels of acculturation. It can be misleading, however, to rely solely on demographic information in this process, especially if the questions or forms used to collect this information are not very specific. For example, in asking for ethnic origin, both a Chinese person and a Japanese person would check the category "Asian"; however, if asked to be specific, they would probably prefer to respond with "Chinese" or "Japanese," respectively. Therefore, although ethnic categories can help identify a cultural group, they do not always provide enough information. One's ethnicity is not necessarily the same as one's culture. People from countries such as China, India, and the Philippines or geographic regions such as Latin America might indicate the same ethnicity (e.g., Chinese, Indian,

Filipino, or Hispanic/Latino) but actually belong to distinct cultural and/or language groups. Therefore, if your program needs to be this specific, you may need to identify languages spoken and the specific traditions in addition to ethnicity.

There are also other distinctions you can make to learn more about your population. For example, if you have identified a large Spanish-speaking population for whom you would like to develop a program, try to find out if they are from the same country or different regions of Latin America. This may be important to know because, though they speak Spanish, some of their health beliefs and practices may be different. Also, depending on their level of acculturation, they may be monolingual or bilingual and have different language preferences. Often older adults will prefer using their native language, whereas teenagers might be more comfortable communicating in English. Also, some may prefer to speak their native language but read and write English. All of this information is relevant and important to consider when developing educational programs and materials for diverse groups.

Therefore, when you are attempting to determine the level of acculturation with respect to the culture you wish to serve, it is helpful to ask questions about language preferences when speaking, reading, and writing, as well as about length of time in the country. Some acculturation scales that were developed for use with different ethnic groups in the United States can be modified to help you with this task. Some of these are listed in the bibliography at the end of the chapter.

Another consideration to help you identify cultural groups is whether patients have common experiences. For example, although both World War II and Vietnam war veterans fought and survived a war, they had very different specific experiences. Therefore they represent two distinct cultural groups and may require very different types of educational programs or services.

TABLE 6.1 Questions to Consider in Gathering Information on a
Target Group's Culture

What name or names do individuals use to define their cultural or ethnic
  identity (e.g., *German, Hispanic, Mexican, Polish, Latino*)?
What is the significance of each name?
What are some major differences between or within cultural groups,
  particularly across generational, educational, socioeconomic, and
  geographical lines?
What are the different education and/or literacy levels within groups? Are
  individuals literate/illiterate in their own language, English, or both?
How many and which languages or dialects are spoken? Is there a common
  language understood by all? Is there a written language?
What type of medical care did they have in their native country?
How is medical care used by these different groups?
What is the expectation for doctors, nurses, and other health professionals?
What are the values of the group or groups you wish to serve?
What are some of the more common health beliefs and practices of the
  various members of different groups?
What are the predominant family structures (hierarchical, patriarchal,
  two-parent household, single-parent household, female-headed household,
  extended, nuclear)?
What are some of the traditional roles of different family members,
  particularly where health is concerned?
Who are the formal and informal leaders in the community, and what role
  do they play with regard to health, health care, and education?
What are the formal and informal channels of communication used by
  your target group?
What are the group's general beliefs about the cause, prevention,
  diagnosis, and treatment of different diseases or health problems?
What are the group's specific beliefs about the health problem that you
  are trying to address?

After you have identified your target groups, you can start
gathering more specific information about the cultures. (Table
6.1 presents a list of some of the questions to consider in your
search.) An easy and more personal approach to gathering this
information is to ask several individuals from the group. For
example, you might ask several patients through informal con-

versations or semistructured interviews. You might also talk with their family members. The bits of information gathered from each patient should help you form a better understanding of some of their cultural beliefs and practices. At the same time, you can reciprocate by sharing with them some of your beliefs and practices. Such exchange promotes the cross-cultural understanding of both provider and patient and helps to build trust and rapport; these are important for the success of your future efforts.

There are also more formal ways of gathering this information from your patient population. These include the use of focus groups and questionnaires. These techniques are discussed in more detail in Chapter 1.

You can also gather information at the library by reading different types of literature about the population to be served. For example, you may want to review historical documents or tapes about the group; these may give you a greater understanding and appreciation for their current circumstances. Also, try to read appropriate medical or public health literature that describes the results of other programs or studies with this population. Behavioral and social science literature, especially ethnic studies or anthropological materials, may provide a general understanding of different cultural beliefs and practices. Finally, read the local newspapers, listen to the radio, or watch television, especially any ethnic newspapers and/or programming targeting the groups you are interested in serving. (If you have never seen local or regional ethnic newspapers, magazines, or programs, this does not mean they do not exist. You may have to hunt to find them. Start by asking your patients; they can be your guides and interpreters, if necessary.) These can give you some insight into the community's problems and concerns and also help you identify people, places, and events to consider later in the development and implementation of your program or services. A reference librarian may also be able to suggest other sources of information.

A third way to gather information is to talk with other people who know something about the community you wish to serve. These might be other professionals working in and with the same community or your friends, colleagues, or coworkers. They can provide yet another perspective about the culture; however, they will be able to report only their own experiences. Also, their experiences may not be representative of the patients you are trying to access, or they may not feel qualified to comment. After all, most of us would feel uncomfortable if asked to describe our own culture.

Finally, try visiting the communities where your patients live. Good community reconnaissance can give you valuable information on how to build a program. Visits should be made at different times of the day on weekdays and weekends so that you can get a good picture of what is happening in the community; this also allows you to be seen. The more time you spend there, the more likely it is that you will become recognized by members of that community.

The best approach in gathering information about your target group is to employ a variety of these methods. In this way, your sources of information will be varied and, it is hoped, less likely to present you with false stereotypes.

¤ HOW DO I CREATE A
CULTURALLY APPROPRIATE PROGRAM?

Creating a culturally appropriate program is no different than creating any other patient education program. You start out with a needs assessment (see Chapter 1), write your objectives (see Chapter 3), and then design a program (see Chapter

3). The only difference is that you take into account and incorporate the appropriate cultural information you learned earlier about the target group. One change in your program might be something as simple as offering the program in a community setting instead of at the hospital or clinic. Or you might have to make more creative changes in the content and process of the program so that it is more relevant. For example, if a group's diet emphasizes certain foods, such as rice and noodles, as staples, then content related to nutrition and/or making dietary changes may need to emphasize these foods rather than potatoes and bread. Also, methods of instruction may need to be modified. For example, if there are varying levels of literacy within the group, you may need to rely on audio- or videotapes rather than written materials for instruction. If the group has definite beliefs about causes of and treatments for certain health problems, then these should be integrated into the teaching.

This is the time to work collaboratively with other people who are bicultural and able to help you make the necessary changes. Ideally, these people should feel very comfortable in both the culture you wish to reach and the majority culture. Although it would also be nice that they have some professional training or expertise in the health field, this is not always possible or realistic. It is important, however, that you, the community, and, it is hoped, your organization trust their cultural expertise. The individuals you identify and choose to work with in the development and implementation of your program must have the trust and respect of the community to ensure the program's credibility and success. One way to gain trust and ensure credibility is to hire individuals from the community to assist with various tasks during different phases of the program's development and implementation.

The success of your program is determined not only by its cultural relevance and the community's acceptance but also by your organization's commitment to serving a culturally diverse population. This commitment to promote cultural diversity is evidenced in how the organization (a) allocates its resources to ensure that quality care and services are both accessible and responsive to the needs of all patients and (b) works to develop collaborative relationships (formal and informal) with different agencies in the ethnic communities it serves. For example, the organization should be committed to recruit and employ not only ancillary staff from the community but also professional staff who can provide clinically, culturally, and linguistically proficient services. Also, your organization might contract services with businesses in that community and endorse or cosponsor community events.

If your organization is not able to make such commitments, it is unlikely that your program will be long lived. Therefore it is important to investigate how and where you might institutionalize your program if it is successful during your planning process. Otherwise, the patients and community may become angry and less willing to work with you or your organization in the future. Lack of commitment and follow-through in the community can adversely affect your reputation and that of your organization.

¤ STRATEGIES FOR ADAPTING PROGRAM CONTENT AND PROCESS

Adapting a program's content and process for different cultures involves more than just translating the information. It also involves the following:

- Changing the actual health information into different, more specific, or more relevant terminology

- Creating new descriptions or explanations that fit better with different people's understanding of key concepts
- Incorporating a group's cultural beliefs and practices into the program content and process

With the help of others, such as an advisory group made up of representatives of the community you wish to serve and/or bilingual, bicultural consultants, review the different sources of information you gathered to identify the culture-specific beliefs and practices about the problem you will address. Use this information to decide how and where to focus the health education efforts. For example, are you interested in providing information to correct certain myths or misconceptions about health, are you attempting to change people's health behaviors, or are you trying to identify and modify some of the environmental factors or barriers that affect health and/or access to health care? Let us examine each of these strategies more closely.

Dispelling Health Misconceptions or Myths

Misconceptions or myths about health, disease, or illness are usually based on incorrect or incomplete information. Therefore one educational strategy might be to correct these misconceptions by helping people reinterpret what they know about the health problem. This can be done by providing more accurate or less confusing explanations about a health problem or by providing new experiences for people to try, helping them reinterpret their understanding of a disease. For example, some individuals or groups believe that arthritis is a fatal disease. This belief is usually based on their own experiences of having seen or known people who suffered greatly with arthritis. They lack complete information about what arthritis is, the types of arthritis, and the importance of treatment to prevent serious problems or complications (e.g., death). Therefore your educational efforts might focus on providing more information about the different types of arthritis and appropriate treatments. As a general rule, when providing this new information, try to limit the use of technical jargon. If you must use technical words, try to explain or define them in lay terms. Also, whenever possible, use visual aids and culturally relevant analogies to help people understand concepts that are complex, abstract, or totally foreign. Another approach might be to help people with arthritis reinterpret what is happening with their disease when they experience changes related to a particular treatment. For example, explain what a specific medication or treatment is doing for them. How is it changing the symptoms they had before? How are they feeling now as a result of the treatment? In this case, the actual experience of the treatment may help to dispel their misconceptions about the disease.

Other misconceptions are formed when people misinterpret the words or messages used to inform them about a disease. For example, some of the misconceptions people have about the transmission of the AIDS virus come from misinterpretations of vague words, such as *bodily fluids,* that were used in early educational campaigns. This vagueness led many people to believe that contact with any or all the body's fluids, including saliva, perspiration, and tears, easily transmitted the virus, which is not the case.

Changing Behavior

Sometimes it is easier to change people's behavior by teaching them new skills than it is to try to change health beliefs and values. People's beliefs and values are usually integral parts of a whole system of understanding (i.e., culture) that are strongly held. Even if a group's beliefs or values seem harmful or unhealthy, they are not likely to change because you point out what is wrong with those beliefs. In fact, doing that would not only be insensitive but alienate the person. Rather, it is best to try to change behaviors by incorporating, not changing, a belief or value.

For example, some ethnic groups believe strongly in the hot-cold theory of disease. The terms *hot* and *cold* do not refer to temperature, but rather to four bodily fluids (sometimes called *humors*) that have certain designations. For example, blood is considered to be hot and wet, yellow bile is hot and dry, phlegm is cold and wet, and black bile is cold and dry. When all these are balanced, the body is healthy; any imbalance causes illness or disease. If a disease is considered hot and wet, the appropriate treatment would have to be the opposite, cold and dry. Therefore, rather than trying to change such an ingrained belief, find out from your patient exactly what foods or medications are considered acceptable treatments for a particular health problem and integrate these into the activities designed to change behaviors. This approach was used by a nutrition educator working with a group of elderly diabetics who believed diabetes was a "hot" disease. In helping them learn how to modify their diets to control the diabetes, she identified foods not only by their nutrients but also by their function. Therefore she was able to emphasize those ethnic foods that were considered "cold" when teaching the elders how to plan their meals. Because she incorporated their belief rather than trying to change it, these elderly were more compliant and better able to control their diabetes through diet.

When culturally adapting activities that encourage behavior change, integrate not only those beliefs or practices specific to health but also others, such as those around food, religion or spirituality, family, music, and exercise. Depending on the cultural group, many of these may be related to perceptions about health as well as health practices.

Changing the Organizational Environment

Patient educators need to work not only with patients to change behaviors but also with the organization to identify and change environmental factors that affect their patients' ability to access appropriate services. In this role, the educator becomes a patient advocate and spokesperson, identifying and suggesting ways the administration might begin to revise policies and procedures so as to value and promote diversity across the board. If the organization can do this in a meaningful way, it may find that more costly services, such as emergency or urgent care, are reduced.

Program Tips

The following are some specific tips to help you begin adapting program content and process for different cultural groups.

1. *Use a multilevel approach.* Making a program more culturally appropriate often means choosing different strategies to tackle different levels of the problem. In this way, the changes achieved are relevant to the individual's health as well as to other aspects of the individual's life (e.g., social, economic conditions, physical environment). For example, a diabetes education program might focus on teaching patients how to make necessary changes in diet and eating habits, while also working with the family to help support these changes and the local community markets to better label or identify healthful food products for people with diabetes.

2. *Do more than translate materials.* Literal translations often result in a product that is inappropriate or even absurd to the target group. It is much better to create new materials from scratch based on the information you have gathered. These can then be pilot-tested on focus groups, who help you to refine the materials. If you need to rely on translated materials, refer to the section on methods of translation later in this chapter.

3. *Incorporate different types of music, art, drama, and/or dance into your patient education activities.* For example, one health department organized a senior theater group whose musical performances demonstrated common medication problems and how seniors might avoid them. The actors were all seniors who represented the ethnic diversity of the community. These plays were given at senior centers and senior housing projects.

4. *Try to personalize the delivery of your program.* Many cultural groups prefer the personal, one-on-one or small-group approaches. Personalizing can be as simple as training staff and volunteers to be warm and friendly with community people, rather than aloof and businesslike. It might also include sending invitations or personalized letters to the people you want to attend, followed up with phone calls as reminders, or encouraging people to call each other during the week as part of the program. Finally, consider a community-based site such as a church or community center rather than the hospital or clinic for the program.

5. *Include different family members as much as possible in the delivery and dissemination of patient education programs.* For example, if elders are the primary source of health advice, train them first to educate others. If you are offering classes, invite family members and significant others to attend. Arrange for transportation and/or child care as needed. When addressing delicate issues such as men's or women's health issues, include activities that educate both sexes about the topics, first separately and then together in groups. For example, a cancer prevention program targeting women might also teach husbands about their wives' need for breast self-examination and

Pap smears. Ideally, as they come to understand why and how these techniques are performed, some men may offer positive support and encouragement for their wives to practice these methods. Or at least, they may no longer interfere with their wives' practice of these methods.

6. *Identify positive role models from the community and train them to deliver your message and/or teach your program.* This method is used frequently in a variety of self-help programs in the health and mental health fields.

7. *Develop health education materials that use clear and simple language to reach people of all educational levels.* There is more information about materials development in Chapter 4.

8. *Ask the community to choose a name for the program so that it has special meaning to them.*

After you have done these things, be sure either to field-test your materials or to run a pilot of your program. Listen for people's comments or watch for their reactions. You may also want to conduct some focus groups to determine whether your ideas and strategies are appropriate and acceptable. They may also provide you with specific suggestions on how to revise your program or materials. Don't be discouraged if you need to make revisions. In fact, be prepared to make at least one revision, if not more, to your program or materials. This does not always mean your attempt was a failure; rather, it means that you are strengthening and improving your work!

¤ TRANSLATION—MORE THAN MEETS THE EYE

If you need to translate materials into other languages, consider carefully the method or methods you choose. Typically, there are three different techniques: one-way translation, translation by committee or consensus, and back-translation (sometimes referred to as *double translation*).

One-Way Translation

One-way translation depends on one bilingual individual to translate the original text into the second language. This is generally the method of choice for most people because it is both simple and economical. The problem with this method is that it assumes that one individual has the necessary comprehensive understanding of both languages and their cultural concepts to make a reliable translation. The mistakes or inaccuracies in the original text are not always identified, and this can lead to possible misinterpretations. Therefore the result is often an awkward literal translation rather than one that represents the real meaning of the text. If you have no choice but to use this method, be sure to have the translation reviewed by other bilingual, bicultural individuals who reflect the diversity within your target group. For example, materials translated into Vietnamese should be reviewed by native speakers from the northern, central, and southern regions of Vietnam to make sure they are easily understood by all. Also, field-test the one-way translation with individuals from the target group and discuss their understanding of the information. These suggestions will help strengthen the quality of a one-way translation.

Translation by Committee or Consensus

This method of translation uses two or more bilingual individuals to translate materials independently. Each translation is then reviewed, and differences are discussed among the translators to produce a consensus version. Because the translation does not rely solely on one individual's knowledge of both languages, the translation is more likely to be accurate. There are, however, some disadvantages to this method. First, it is more time consuming and less economical. Also, if the translators do not reflect the diversity from within the community you are trying to reach, the translation may not be appropriate. For example, if you choose only professionals to translate, the translated material may be too difficult for your patients to understand or may not represent the vernacular of this group. In fact, this is a common problem even when you are writing in the same language. Finally, when trying to reach consensus, some of the translators may not feel comfortable contributing their ideas about the appropriateness of the translation. That is, one translator may defer to members of the committee who are older or more educated, but not necessarily right. Therefore your translation may appear to be a consensus version but actually conceal real disagreements about meaning. These limitations, however, can be avoided by (a) choosing a diverse group of translators from the target community and (b) allowing each to provide you with his or her written comments about the different translations prior to the consensus meeting. You or someone else can then facilitate the discussion about any noted disagreements. You may also want another person to review the consensus version and/or field-test it with some of your patients.

Back-Translation

Back-translation requires at least two translators working independently. One translates the original material into the second language; the other takes this translated material and translates it back into the original language. The two original-language versions are then compared to identify significant differences. These differences are then discussed with the translators to determine the better alternative, or another round of back-translations can be done. This method has several advantages despite being more costly and time consuming. First, it allows for more than one interpretation of both the language and cultural concepts, thereby producing a more appropriate translation. This is especially so if more than one round of translations is done. Translators can meet to discuss differences in translation and any problems with regard to cultural relevance. Second, this method encourages each translator to treat his or her version as the original and discourages him or her from trying to infer meaning or make sense of a poor translation. At the time that each translator receives the material, ask each to identify words that could be translated in different ways or have different meanings, as well as any words or phrases that are awkward or nonsensical when translated. This allows you to consider alternative wording if regional differences exist in the second language. Again, the final translation should be field-tested. After the translation has been used and refined, consider modifying the original material so that it is linguistically more equivalent to the translated version. By doing this, you may improve the original text by making it less ambiguous in meaning or more easily understood. (Table 6.2 lists some tips on writing translatable English.)

The back-translation method is really the most reliable because it allows you to see the differences between the original and back-translated versions of the material. These differences, in turn, show you not only how the material has been translated but also how it has been adapted so that it is culturally relevant.

TABLE 6.2 Tips on Writing Translatable English

Use simple language from the outset (grade-school level).

Use nouns rather than pronouns.

Avoid the use of metaphors or colloquial expressions (it is difficult to
   translate these and maintain the proper connotation).

Avoid possessive forms of words that may be misinterpreted when more
   than one actor is involved.

Use specific rather than general terms.

Avoid words that indicate vagueness about an event.

Use short and simple sentences (i.e., fewer than 16 words).

Use the active rather than the passive voice.

Avoid the subjunctive (e.g., verb forms with *would* or *could*).

Avoid adverbs and prepositions telling when and where (unless specific).

Avoid sentences with two different verbs if the verbs suggest different
   actions.

Use redundant wording to clarify the context and meaning of a phrase.

¤ CONCLUSION

The creation of culturally relevant patient education programs is not an easy task, but can be interesting and rewarding.
We hope that the suggestions we have discussed in this chapter
will help you approach this task more confidently, knowing that
it involves careful research, planning, and, if possible, the
collaboration of different people, especially the individuals you
want to serve. It is their input that ensures the program's
relevance and success. Though the suggestions presented here
cannot guarantee your program's success, they certainly improve your chances for success and can help you establish a
better working relationship with the different cultural groups
in the future.

¤ BIBLIOGRAPHY

American Hospital Association. (1982). *Culture-bound and sensory barriers to communication with patients: Strategies and resources for health education.* Springfield, VA: National Technical Information Service.

Brownlee, A. (1978). *Community, culture, and care: A cross-cultural guide for health workers.* Saint Louis, MO: Mosby.

Burnam, M. A., Telles, C. A., Karno, M., Hough, R. L., & Escobar, J. I. (1987). Measurement of acculturation in a community population of Mexican Americans. *Hispanic Journal of Behavioral Sciences, 9,* 105-130.

Deyo, R. A., Diehl, A. K., Hazuda, H., & Stern, M. P. (1985). A simple language-base acculturation scale for Mexican Americans: Validation and application to health care research. *American Journal of Public Health, 75,* 51-55.

Gonzalez, V. M., Gonzalez, J. T., Freeman, V., & Howard-Pitney, B. (1991). *Health promotion in diverse cultural communities.* Stanford, CA: Stanford University Press.

Harwood, A. (Ed.). (1981). *Ethnicity and medical care.* Cambridge, MA: Harvard University Press.

Henderson, G., & Primeaux, M. (Eds.). (1981). *Transcultural health care.* Menlo Park, CA: Addison-Wesley.

Marin, G., & Marin, B. V. (1991). *Research with Hispanic populations.* Newbury Park, CA: Sage.

Marin, G., Sabogal, F., Marin, B. V., Otero-Sabogal, R., & Perez-Stable, E. J. (1987). Development of a short acculturation scale for Hispanics. *Hispanic Journal of Behavioral Sciences, 9,* 183-205.

Orque, M., Block, B., & Monrroy, L. (1983). *Ethnic nursing care: A multicultural approach.* Saint Louis, MO: Mosby.

Padilla, A. M. (Ed.). (1980). *Acculturation: Theory, models and some new findings.* Boulder, CO: Westview.

Randall-David, E. (1989). *Strategies for working with culturally diverse communities and clients.* Washington, DC: Association for the Care of Children's Health.

7

Helping People Who Are Hard to Help

Kate Lorig

One of the greatest challenges in patient education is dealing with people who are hard to help. Fortunately, there are a limited number of problems that seem to appear over and over again. Once you recognize them and their solutions, dealing with them becomes much easier. In this chapter, you will meet some of the most common types of problem people and learn ways of helping them.

¤ STRONG, SILENT TYPES

One of the greatest fears of patient educators is that they will not be able to get people to ask questions or to discuss topics. There is also a strongly held belief that "people here are different. They don't talk." "Here" can mean any region, country, or culture.

People are not really all that different. Rather, it is the patient educators who are insecure about their own knowledge and abilities and never really invite participation. Usually they give a talk and then ask if there are any questions. Given 10 seconds and no response, they decide that there are no questions and continue or end the session.

If you are trying to get participation, several techniques will be very helpful. You might present a problem or question, such as "What would you do if. . . ?" Have all the participants write down their answers. Then go around the room, having each participant tell what he or she wrote. This technique ensures that everyone participates in a nonthreatening way. But in using this technique, first be sure that the question is one that is nonthreatening and with which the participants have experience—for example, "What is the greatest problem in controlling your diet?" When using this technique, the leader should start by modeling an appropriate response using a personal experience. Finally, start with a participant who you know will be able to respond. Once the group is clear on the expectation and knows that responses will be handled in a nonjudgmental way, generally everyone will follow.

A second way of getting group participation is to brainstorm. The details for this technique are discussed in Chapter 3 in the section "Brainstorming."

When asking the group questions, be sure that the question is open-ended. A good rule to follow is never to ask a question that can be answered by *yes* or *no.* "What questions do you have?" is better than "Are there any questions?" Then, after asking for questions, count to 30 slowly. Groups do not like silence, and someone will generally say something to fill the void. If the silence makes you uncomfortable, you can add a second prompt such as "Surely there are some questions?" Once the ice is broken, more questions and discussion usually follow.

Make the group safe for questions and discussions. Give reinforcement to everyone who participates, with smiles, nods of your head, or positive comments such as "That is a good question" or "I'm so glad you asked that. Many people have the same problem and are afraid to discuss it." Be careful not to make participants feel stupid or silly. Even if you get a bizarre comment, respond with a noncommittal, neutral statement such as "That's an interesting comment" or "I see your point of view."

By using the above techniques, you can almost always get good group participation. However, there may still be some nonparticipating group members. First, be sure that these people are sitting in the group. Often they will place themselves physically outside the group. If someone is a chronic nonparticipant, address questions directly to him or her—for example, "Jim/Maria, what do you think about that?" Be sure that you do not put the nonparticipant on the spot. Always ask something that you know he or she can answer.

Sometimes you will have situations in which husbands or wives answer for their spouses or parents answer for their child. In these cases, address your questions directly to the child or silent spouse. If someone else answers, say, "No, let Jill speak for herself." Then be patient and let this happen. Be especially sure to reinforce any participation by your strong, silent types. In addition, watch them carefully for any sign that they might like to participate but are holding back. A change in posture or facial expression or a slightly raised finger may be all the clue you get. Do not miss these.

In almost every class you will have a sleeper. Do not let this worry you. Just let the person sleep. He or she is probably tired. It has nothing to do with your presentation. If more than 25% of the class is sleeping, then you might be the problem. However, if the class is made up of medical students or doctors, even a 50% sleep rate is acceptable.

¤ TALKERS

Once you have gotten your group to participate, the problem will probably be shutting them up. Too much participation can be just as bad as no participation; this takes skill to control. Here are some situations that might arise.

Participants come to a course with some special problems or question. They often want these answered right away. As a leader, you can easily be thrown from your agenda by trying to meet participants' needs immediately. Do not be afraid to say, "We are going to discuss medications in the third session. Right now we are discussing exercise" or "That is a little off the topic, but I will be pleased to discuss it with you over coffee. Right now it is important to get on with the class." To help keep this situation from occurring, you should have an agenda posted at the start of each class, divided into topics and with the time allowed. Then, if you are behind, you can use the agenda as a reason for charging ahead.

One of the most troublesome of all class participants is the talker. He or she almost always has something to say, which usually includes a long story. Sometimes the stories and insights are useful and relevant, and other times they are useless. In either case, the person who usurps time must be controlled.

One way to do this is just not to call on the person. But this is of limited usefulness as this person will often butt in, asked or not. Sometimes you have to be very blunt: "Your opinions are helpful, but others need a chance to be heard." This may seem harsh and unfeeling; however, such a statement is usually handled with good grace. The people who hog time know when they are being "hoggish." Sometimes you can use the seating arrangement to control this situation. If you sit next to the talker, it is more difficult for him or her to get your attention and cut in.

Another frequent problem is when a participant rambles on and on. The point of the story, if there is a point, was made in the first 15 seconds. In this case, the only thing to do is cut the person off. Wait until he or she takes a breath—it has to happen sometime—and quickly say, "Thank you very much." Immediately call on someone else or start a new activity. At the same time, physically turn away from the person.

Side talkers are very common. These are people who are always chatting to their neighbors. To begin with, ask them to be quiet. If this does not work, sit between the two friends. This is sometimes successful. If not, a little sarcasm might be helpful: "If you two don't stop talking, I'll have to ask one of you to stand in the corner."

There is one special case of talker. People who arrive late almost always try to "make up" for their lateness by immediate participation. This participation may be inappropriate or even destructive. You can sidetrack this a bit by helping to integrate the person. For example, "Joe, we were worried about you. I'm glad you're here. We were just discussing. . . ."

On very rare occasions, you will find a whole class that is very difficult to control. They all talk at once. In this case, seating can come to your rescue. Although we generally like to have small groups sit in a circle, sitting people in rows, in desks, or with tables in front of them tends to reestablish control and quiet discussion. If all else fails, rearrange the room. Of course, if the problem is lack of participation in a formal setting, try making the setting less formal.

¤ ANTAGONISTIC OR BELLIGERENT PARTICIPANTS

Fortunately, these people do not appear too often. They, too, can be helped. The first thing to remember is not to argue. This just leads to more argument. Instead, try "I understand your beliefs but our current knowledge in this suggests . . ." or "If you find eating fish cures your ulcers, then please continue eating fish. However, for most people we find that _____ will be more helpful."

Sometimes a leader and a participant will argue with each other. Somehow, whatever the leader says adds more antagonism. When this happens, it is usually a play for power from someone who is used to being the center of attention. One way to help this situation is to place the powermonger out of direct eye contact. In a circle, the best way of doing this is to place the person next to the leader. Somehow, being out of eye contact tends to defuse the situation.

If all else fails, you may have to ask the belligerent person to leave the class. This can be done by saying, "I don't think this class will meet your needs. If you will see me during coffee or call me tomorrow, we can see if we can find something more suitable." At this point the belligerent person may leave. More likely, he or she will simmer down and participate more appropriately. In either case, things will be easier for you and for participants.

¤ "YES, BUTS"

These are the people who always have an excuse for not doing what you ask. They are usually easy to identify by their distinctive call "Yes, but. . . ." After hearing two or three "yes, buts," give up. An easy rule of thumb is, three "yes, buts" and they are out. There is no way you can help them by being helpful. Instead, confront them:

> I know that you have many problems. However, the decision to do something or not is yours. I do not have high blood pressure, so it is not my problem. If you want to do something, fine; I will try to be helpful. If not, that is okay too. It is your choice.

Such a statement makes it very clear where the problem lies and that it is up to the individual to take responsibility. Do not spend all your time with these people. You probably will not be able to help them. In trying to help them, you deny help to others who are more ready to act. One of the best ways of turning a "Yes, But" around is to ignore him or her. Often, when someone gets attention for action rather than nonaction, you see a change in his or her behavior.

The "Know-It-All" is just a variation of the "Yes, But." This person knows all the answers and has tried everything. There is nothing you can teach him or her. Acknowledge that the person is very knowledgeable and that you might not be able to teach him or her anything. Then give him or her the choice of continuing or leaving. Most of the time, once the game is called, the person will become an active and helpful participant. Sometimes he or she will leave, and this is okay too.

¤ ATTENTION SEEKERS

We have already talked about several types of attention seekers—the Belligerents, the "Know-It-Alls," and the "Yes, Buts." There are two more types, which, unfortunately, have a high prevalence in patient education classes.

The Whiners are those people with a million problems. Sometimes they are also "Yes, Buts." Somehow they manage to get the whole class involved in the catastrophe they call life. Everyone feels sorry for them. Often their stories are truly traumatic—they were molested as children, have alcoholic husbands, or are about to get evicted from the family home. Besides, no one loves them. First, you must remember that the story may or may not be true. Second, there are probably three or four other people in the class with equally wrenching lives who somehow are coping and productive. If you and the class get bogged down with whiners, no one wins and everyone loses. Instead, suggest that you will talk with them at coffee or after class and try to make some appropriate referrals. Do not spend class time in trying to solve their problems!

The second group of attention seekers play a game called "My disease is worse than your disease." They seek status by having the worst disease. It is important to cut this game short at the beginning. Statements such as the following may help:

In this class everyone has problems with _____. Some of these may seem worse than others, but you can never judge another by your standard. The paraplegic in a loving family may get along very well, while the loss of a finger can be devastating to a concert violinist. In this class we will try to help everyone with his or her problems and not make judgments about the severity of the problems.

Another way of cutting short this disease status game is not to let participants give their disease history or to describe themselves in terms of the disease. This is especially important in introductions. Ask people to tell about their families, hobbies, or what they want to get out of the course or the problems caused by their condition. *Do not ask* them to tell about their disease.

¤ SPECIAL PROBLEM PEOPLE

Two final types of problem people are not very common but need to be recognized and dealt with quickly: the "ists" and the "inappropriates."

The "ists" are the people who are racists, sexists, or ageists. They are the men who call women "girls," the young people who make rude remarks about older people, and those who use terms such as *niggers* and *Japs*. Any time you encounter an "ist," you should make it clear that such language and thinking do not have a place in this setting. This is true even if you do not have Asians or older people in your class.

In some ways, the "inappropriates" are the easiest to handle. These are the people who clearly have a mental health problem that is usually obvious in the first few minutes of the class. If their speech and behavior is not disruptive, then let them stay. However, if they are in any way disruptive, then help them find a more appropriate setting to work on their problems. It is not fair to the rest of the class to keep such a person around. Again, everyone, including the inappropriate person, loses.

This chapter has discussed the most common problem people. Sometimes you may encounter other problems or a group of people with multiple problems. In this case, seek some help. A psychologist or social worker who has experience with group work can be an excellent resource. When you are in trouble, do not be afraid to ask for help.

8

The Special Problem of Compliance
How Do I Get People to Do What Is Good for Them?

Kate Lorig

V arious authors and studies have estimated that people comply with new health behaviors 30% to 70% of the time. On face value, this paints a sorry picture and suggests that compliance is a major problem. However, it is necessary to examine this issue a bit more closely.

For some health-related regimes, compliance is a very important issue. We know that it is necessary for many people to take insulin daily in order to control diabetes. However, we do not have any similar data to suggest the exact type, amount, or duration of exercise necessary either to prevent or to overcome the musculoskeletal problems caused by arthritis. Much of arthritis is physical therapy practice, common sense, and clinical experience. However, it is not backed by strong scientific evidence. When such evidence is lacking, it is difficult to justify the importance of exact compliance with an exercise program.

Another issue involves the interactions between the disease and the desired health behaviors. For many diseases, the symptoms wax and wane on almost a daily basis. Therefore the lock-step continuation of a set of behaviors in the face of changing symptoms does not seem to make a great deal of sense. Rather than demonstrating strict compliance, a person must understand the rationale for his or her program and also know how to make daily adjustments in the face of these changing symptoms. If this is not done, behavior change becomes a frustrating experience in which the patient either exacerbates the symptoms or gets no therapeutic effect because the intervention is not tailored to the symptoms. Balancing behavior change with symptoms takes knowledge, practice, and, most important, decision-making skills. Unfortunately, health professionals seldom teach decision-making skills in traditional interactions with patients.

On the basis of the above discussion, it would seem that specific compliance may not always be a desired or even a necessary behavior. A more appropriate goal might be adherence to a long-term program with constant changes in response to symptoms. However, even with this broader definition, it is doubtful that most people would adopt new programs appropriately. The rest of this chapter will discuss reasons for inappropriate compliance patterns, ways of identifying problems with individual patients, and suggestions for solving these problems. The terms *compliance* and *adherence* will be used interchangeably.

Let us now turn to exploring how to help people with compliance. This will be done with the decision chart in Figure 8.1. Start at the top and work through until you find a description

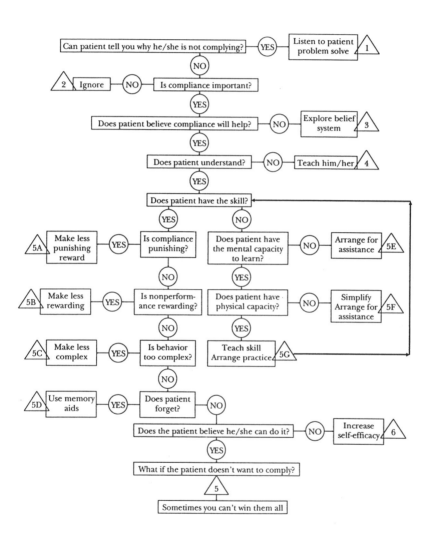

Figure 8.1. Improving Patient Compliance

of the problem you are encountering. Each level of the chart lists one or more actions that might be taken in the boxes next to the triangles. Look up further discussion of these actions in the text that follows by seeking the number (or number and letter) that is given in the triangle.

1. *Can the patient tell you why he or she is not complying?*

This may seem like an obvious question. However, all too often we forget to ask. When we do ask, the patient will usually tell us the problem. The normal response of most professionals when confronted with a patient problem is to offer the patient a solution. This is probably not the best response. Rather, this is an ideal time to teach problem-solving skills. To do this, ask the patient to brainstorm possible solutions. For example, if a patient says she does not have enough time to exercise in the morning, ask when else in the day she might have 10 minutes to do her exercises. If a patient says he forgets to exercise, ask about activities that he does daily, such as reading the morning paper or watching a favorite TV show, and then link the exercises to one such activity. The moral here is that most patients can tell you the problem and, with a little assistance, come up with a solution. Never underestimate your patient.

2. *Is compliance important?*

This may seem like a silly question. However, as discussed earlier, we really do not know exactly which exercise program is best for which patient. The result is that we often ask patients to do things that may not be important. For example, are daily range-of-motion exercises necessary for every stroke patient? The answer is probably no. In fact, range-of-motion exercise three or four times a week is probably sufficient. Do all joints need to be put through a daily range-of-motion exercise?

Again, the answer is probably no. One needs to exercise only those joints in which there is some limitation. If compliance is not important, then forget about it. Both you and the patient have more important things to worry about.

3. *Does your patient believe that compliance will help?* (No).

If the answer is no, then the reason for noncompliance is obvious. Why should anyone do anything in which he or she does not believe? Although the problem may be obvious, the solution is a bit more difficult. People's beliefs are almost always rational and based on culture, past experience, conversations with others, and/or what they have been taught. Often it is the use of language that leads patients to false beliefs. Arthritis health professionals often talk about osteoarthritis as a "wear-and-tear disease." It is not. When heard by patients, this idea is easily translated into rational action: "Why should I exercise if my disease is caused by wear and tear? Exercise increases the problem." One of the ways to help to change beliefs is to change the use of language. Avoid using the incorrect "wear-and-tear" explanation for osteoarthritis.

Another means of changing beliefs is to expand on the patient's current belief system. If someone believes that pain is due to disease, then the way to counter the pain is through medical interventions such as medication. However, if this explanation of pain is expanded to include not only disease but also muscle tension, fear, and depression, then other pain management modalities, such as exercise and relaxation, may be tried.

Finding out patients' beliefs is not difficult—ask them. Good questions include "What do you think causes your pain?" "Why is exercise important?" and "When you think of diabetes, what do you think of?" Before giving any explanation, it is important to find out what the patient already knows and believes. In this way, teaching is targeted and time is not wasted (more about beliefs in Chapter 1, the section "Salient Beliefs Assessment").

4. *Does the patient understand?* (No).

Do not believe that patients understand just because they say they do. This is especially true with medication regimes. It is one thing to repeat what the doctor says and quite another to integrate medication taking into one's regime. If people are not sure of what they are doing, they will often do nothing rather than risk doing something wrong. Another problem is that we often give instructions only for the ideal case—for example, "Take this medication twice a day." We do not tell patients what to do in real cases—for example, "If you miss one dose, take it as soon as you remember. Do not double up doses."

Whenever you give patients instructions, take four steps to ensure understanding. First, tell patients what you want them to do in plain English. Forget all the terms such as *TID*. Second, if you want patients to exercise, show them what you want them to do and have them return the demonstration until they can do so easily without coaching. Third, give patients written instructions, including, if necessary, pictures. Finally, ask patients to describe what they are going to do. Do not accept a parroting of your original explanation. Rather, ask questions such as "When are you going to take your medicine, and how many pills will you take each time?" In short, TWA—tell, write, ask.

5. *Does the patient have the skill to comply?* (Yes).

5A. *Is compliance punishing?* (Yes).

In many cases, complying with health regimes is not only nonrewarding but punishing. For example, many drugs have side effects, diets take away pleasures, and exercise may leave one stiff. Each of these cases is a bit different, but the solution is similar: Make compliance less punishing and more rewarding. When compliance means physiological punishment, such as stiffness from exercise, symptom reinterpretation is useful. (See more about this in Chapter 9, the section "Reinterpretation of Physiological Signs and Symptoms.") Explain that the stiffness means that the treatment is actually doing some good. The patient might interpret stiffness as meaning that the exercise is causing worsening of the disease.

In another case, exercise might be punishing because of the time of day or weather conditions. Few people like to walk a mile on a cold winter day before breakfast. In this case, another time might be found, or a warm place such as a shopping mall, or even an alternate exercise, such as riding a stationary bicycle.

5B. *Is nonperformance rewarding?* (Yes).

Sometimes noncompliance brings rewards such as attention, albeit nagging, from spouses or friends. Also, the short-term rewards of noncompliance, such as remaining in bed on a cold morning, might outweigh the long-term rewards of a daily early morning walk. If noncompliance is rewarding, the best thing to do is to remove the reward. Ignoring noncompliance may be difficult but may also be the best way to bring about improvement. This is especially true with couples in which sometimes the only communication is nagging. Reestablishing more positive communication patterns may be the answer.

5C. *Is the behavior too complex?* (Yes).

Sometimes we ask patients to do many things all at the same time. They are taking several medications, are on a special diet, and have three sets of exercises to perform daily. In addition, they are asked to have appointments with one or more health professionals on a regular basis. Is it any wonder that they do not comply? Before talking to patients about compliance, it is important to get the whole picture of what they are trying to do. Ask them, "What are all the things that various people have told you to do?" These may range from flossing teeth to drinking warm milk before going to bed every night. What you want them to do is only a small part of the total picture and, compared with some other activities, may be relatively unimportant. In any case, as a health professional, you have the job of sorting out the jumble and simplifying the regime. This may mean contacting other health professionals to see which of their instructions are really important. In some cases, the instructions may even be contradictory. For example, the rheumatologist says to limit weight-bearing exercise because of bad knees, but the cardiologist says to forget the knees and walk as much as possible. The patient loses no matter what he or she does. Once one understands the whole regime, priorities can be set and complexities simplified.

5D. *Does the patient forget?* (Yes).

This is probably one of the greatest causes of noncompliance. It is not easy to add a new activity to our lives, especially if this activity must be performed more than once a day. Memory aids, such as setting an alarm clock or wristwatch, can remind one when it is time to take medications. Medicine bottles can now be purchased with built-in alarms.

Another and more powerful memory aid is to link the new behavior with an already established activity. For example, range-of-motion exercises can be done in the morning shower, and a walk can be taken before lunch. Medication can be taken when brushing teeth. Most of us are creatures of habit. The easiest way to establish a new habit is to link it with an existing habit. Those who are cognitively impaired may need more help. A sample of all pills and the times they are to be taken can be posted on a board. Then the day's pills can be laid out below the sample. The patient needs only to look at the board to find out if he or she has taken the pill. Using this method, the patient might be able to lay out his or her own pills each day.

5E. *Does the patient have the mental capacity to learn the skill?* (No).

If the answer is no, you might try some of the tricks under memory aids. However, it is more likely that you will need to find someone to assist the patient. This might be a spouse or other family member, a neighbor, or possibly a home health aide or visiting PT. Many older people who live alone are part of an informal helping network of friends and neighbors. Such networks are especially helpful for the cognitively impaired. Is there someone who can call twice a day to remind the patient to do something? Maybe there is a neighbor who will take a daily walk with the patient or assist with medication taking. In any case, the answer is usually to find some assistance.

5F. *Does the patient have the physical capacity to do the skill?* (No).

If the answer is no, then there are several routes to take. First, the activity might be simplified or changed to bring it within the physical capacity of the patient. See 5C for suggestions on how to make activities less complex. On the other hand, the patient may need assistance. The suggestions under 5E might be helpful.

5G. *Teach skill and arrange practice and feedback.*

If the patient does not have the skill but has the cognitive and physical capacity to learn the skill, then the tricks to compliance are teaching, practice, and feedback. First, the patient must be taught the skill. This can sometimes be done verbally or in writing. However, if there is any unusual physical skill involved, then teaching must include demonstration and practice. One cannot learn to ride a bicycle from reading a book. It is not realistic to expect patients to learn to inject insulin from written materials. Rather, patients need an opportunity for supervised practice and feedback. It is especially important that during the demonstration patients do the whole activity without assistance. This may be very frustrating for the health professional. However, the important thing is that patients leave the teaching session confident that they can "do it themselves." Remember that even the most complex behavior can be broken down into simple, achievable parts.

The final part of teaching a skill is arranging for feedback. This can be provided as part of the demonstration/return demonstration. Compliance is even more likely if patients have a way of getting their questions answered and receiving feedback when they are at home. This can often be provided by telephone. Another possibility is sending patients home with a video so that they can review the procedure.

6. *Does the patient believe that he or she can do it?* (No).

This is probably the key to many compliance problems. Just because people know how to do something and even have the required skills does not mean they believe they can do it. Many people who are overweight believe that this condition is harmful, know all about exercise and low-calorie food, and even know how to exercise and eat appropriately. However, all these beliefs and knowledge are not enough, because these people do not believe themselves capable of carrying out the program and losing weight. Bandura (1982) called this belief in one's ability to carry out specific behaviors *perceived self-efficacy*. In this case, your job is to increase the patient's confidence. See the section on self-efficacy in Chapter 9.

7. *What if the patient does not want to comply?*

Just because you want patients to do something and know that it is good for them is no reason they have to agree. Patients have a right to make their own decisions for their own reasons. You should be convinced that the decision is informed. That is, patients understand your rationale for wanting them to do something. Once this criterion is met, if patients still decide not to comply, you should honor their decision. Health professionals have a limited amount of time. Often time is wasted trying to work with patients who have no intention of changing. More important, it deprives other patients who can be helped of the health professional's time. Sometimes the best thing to do is to just let a patient go. If this occurs, make very clear what you are doing. The conversation might go something like this: "Mrs. Jones, I understand that you do not want to exercise. We have discussed the various reasons that exercise might be good for you. However, I do respect your decision. If in the future I can help you with an exercise program, please let me know." This conversation does several things. First, it lets Mrs. Jones know that the decision not to exercise is hers. Second, it leaves the door open should she change her mind. Finally, it shows your respect for her, even though you disagree with her decision.

In short, if people do not want to comply, you cannot make them. Sometimes you just cannot win them all.

¤ BIBLIOGRAPHY

Bandura, A. (1982). Self-efficacy in human agency. *American Psychologist, 37,* 122-147.

Cramer, J. A., & Spilder, B. (Eds.). (1991). *Patient compliance in medical practice and clinical trials.* New York: Raven.

Mager, R. F., & Pipe, P. (1970). *Analyzing performance problems.* Belmont, CA: Fearon.

Sackett, D. L., & Haynes, R. B. (1976). *Compliance with therapeutic regimes.* Baltimore: Johns Hopkins University Press.

9

What We Know About What Works
One Rationale, Two Models, Three Theories

Jean Goeppinger
Kate Lorig

Patient education, at least good patient education, does not just happen. Rather, it is planned with the use of a rationale and one or more models and/or theories. In this chapter we examine an overall rationale for patient education, two commonly used models, and three theories. These have been selected because they seem especially applicable to patient education. Before beginning, let us define terms. A *rationale* is a statement of *reasons, models* are *plans* or ways of organizing things, and *theories* are systems of ideas used to *explain changes* such as improved behaviors or health.

Before going further, one must understand why all of this is important. Models and theories do not tell us exactly what to do. They do not work in the same way in all situations. Rather, they serve as guidelines for practice. The more you know about models and theories, the more tools you will have for building strong, successful patient education interventions. An analogy might be helpful. It is difficult to impossible to build a house with your bare hands. But with basic tools such as a hammer and a saw, and some practice in using them, the task becomes easier. As you add more tools and more practice, you can build ever more complex and useful houses. So it is with patient education. It is difficult to build a successful program without theory. Good programs are built using a combination of models and theories. Just as there are many tools, there are many models and theories.

The models and theories that appear in this chapter were chosen because they seem especially applicable to patient education. That is, they help to plan for complex situations and complex change. They also apply to much of health promotion, in which we are usually trying to change only one or two behaviors at a time. Once you become familiar with these tools and begin to use them, you will find that you do not always have the right model or theory for the task at hand. This is no reason to give up on theory. Rather, it is a reason for learning more. The bibliography at the end of the chapter should be helpful. You might also want to subscribe to *Patient Education and Counseling* or *Health Education Quarterly*.[1] These publications are very useful for learning more about the theory and practice of patient education.

¤ RATIONALE: THE COMPRESSION OF MORBIDITY

In 1981, Fries and Crapo published their book *Vitality and Aging*, in which they argued that the human life span is finite. That is, no matter what improvements we make, the average human being will probably not live more than 85 to 95 years. The future will not produce 200-year-old people. If this is true, then the purpose of all health care is to reduce premature morbidity and mortality. Fries and Crapo (1981) termed this *rectangularizing the curve*. Some examples will clarify this further.

At the present time, someone is born and, barring anything unusual, lives a fairly healthy life until well into the fifth or sixth decade. At this point, he or she may encounter any of a number of chronic illnesses: hypertension, diabetes, heart disease, osteoporosis, or arthritis, to name just a few. These illnesses take away from quality of life. The person's health generally declines for the next 15 to 30 years until death (see Figure 9.1).

To say that we are going to prevent death from heart disease or diabetes may be unrealistic. However, we may be able to compress morbidity. That is, instead of having a situation in which people get diseases at age 60 and live with chronic problems for the next 20 years, we may be able to push the onset of disease back to age 75, thus compressing the morbidity. Even when someone has an illness, such as heart disease or hypertension, we may be able to stabilize the condition rather than have it progress on a steady downward path. Again, this compresses morbidity (see Figure 9.2). Thus the rationale for health promotion and patient education is to allow people to live the fullest life possible for the longest possible time and to compress the time that they are infirm due to ill health. Now that we have a reason for doing patient education, let us examine some theories and how they might be applied to real-world practice.

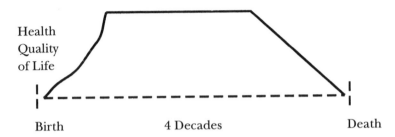

Figure 9.1. Natural "Life History" of Morbidity at Present

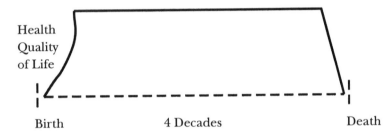

Figure 9.2. Natural "Life History" of Morbidity Projected as a Goal of Health Education

¤ THREE THEORIES: SELF-EFFICACY, STRESS AND COPING, AND LEARNED HELPLESSNESS

The purpose of a theory is to provide an explanation of why things happen. If this explanation is accurate, then if we do things a second time, the result should be the same as the first. Theories make the world a much less chaotic place. For example, if we drop a plate, it will fall and probably break. Knowing this, we do not have to keep dropping plates to see what happens. The same is true in patient education. Our theories are far from perfect, but we do know some things. For example,

Houland (1957) taught us that when we are trying to persuade someone of something, it is better to give both sides of the argument, instead of just one. Earlier we discussed how salient belief theory can be useful in needs assessments (see Chapter 1). In short, the wise use of theory helps us make things happen. There is no need for each new patient educator to drop a dozen plates or run a dozen programs before being horrified with the results.

Many theories can be applied to patient education. These come from the fields of communication, organizational development, sociology, psychology, and adult education. The best patient education is an appropriate mix and match of theory. This mixing and matching, like being a good cook, comes from experience. However, one cannot mix and match without knowing what exists. The three theories to be discussed here were chosen because they have particular relevance to patient education.

Self-Efficacy Theory

According to Bandura (personal communication, 1992; see also Bandura, 1982, 1986),

> Perceived self-efficacy theory states that: 1) The state of belief in one's ability is a good predictor of motivation and behavior. 2) In addition one's self-efficacy beliefs can be enhanced through performance mastery, modeling, reinterpretation of physiological symptoms and social persuasion. 3) Finally, enhanced self-efficacy leads to improved behaviors, motivation, thinking patterns and emotional well being. It is not concerned with the skills one has but with judgments of what one can do with whatever skills one possesses.

Several parts of this definition need emphasis. First, self-efficacy is behavior-specific. That is, there is no such thing as an efficacious person. Rather, someone may have very high efficacy for getting dressed in the morning but very low efficacy for flying an airplane. In this way, self-efficacy differs from two related constructs: learned helplessness and locus of control (Seligman, 1975; Wallston, Wallston, Kaplan, & Maides, 1976). Learned-helplessness theory suggests that when people feel they have no control over their lives, as in the case of an unpredictable chronic illness, the result is an increased feeling of helplessness, which most often manifests as depression (for more on learned helplessness, see the section later in this chapter). Locus-of-control theory examines how people see their lives being controlled. Some people feel that most of the control is in their own hands. These people are likely to work hard at making changes in behaviors that they believe will help them. Other people feel that control is external. In such cases, the doctor, God, or some other force controls their lives. These people are likely to feel that there is nothing they can do to help their situation. Both locus of control and learned helplessness are generalized to one's whole being and are not behavior-specific.

Second, self-efficacy deals with one's perception or belief that one can accomplish some future behavior. In this way it is predictive. One's efficacy for future performance is a good predictor of actual future performance. Thus, if I were a circus owner who had to employ a new unicycle rider immediately and could not test applicants' skills, I would ask potential employees how certain they were that, given some brief instruction, they could ride a unicycle. I would then choose the applicant with the highest efficacy, as he or she would be most likely to master quickly the art of unicycle riding.

On the other hand, sometimes there are people who perform quite well but believe that their performance is not up to standard. These people have low efficacy, which, in turn, may prevent them from trying anything more challenging.

Finally, research has shown us that we can change self-efficacy and that changes in self-efficacy are associated with changes in behavior and cognitive states such as pain and stress. Thus, if we enhance someone's efficacy for not smoking, he or she is more likely not to smoke. Because of all these characteristics, self-efficacy theory has great applicability to patient education (Bandura, 1982).

There are four specific efficacy-enhancing mechanisms: (a) skills mastery, (b) modeling, (c) reinterpretation of physiological signs and symptoms, and (d) social persuasion.

Skills Mastery

Probably the most powerful way of enhancing self-efficacy is through skills mastery. This is generally done by breaking skills into very small, manageable tasks and then making sure that each small task is successfully completed. Some of the original work was done with agoraphobics who first walked outside their door, then walked a few steps, then walked to the sidewalk, and so on. Another good example is Alcoholics Anonymous, in which members promise not to drink today. They do not worry about tomorrow. In other words, each commitment or contract is short-term, not for life. In devising health education programs, we have found that it is best to have people start with what they are sure they can do now. For example, the person who has had a stroke and who can walk half a block is encouraged to do this four times a week and then add to the program by no more than 10% each week. Remember that the key to skills mastery is the word *mastery*. If people are going to become more efficacious, it is important that they be successful in what they are trying to do.

One of the best ways of accomplishing mastery is to have clients contract for specific behaviors. Contracting should be mostly client driven. That is, the individual decides on the behavior; it is not dictated by the professional. Equally important, there must be an opportunity to give feedback and make mid-course corrections. Every session of a health education course might end with a contracting session, and every session might begin with feedback for the past week. This point is so important that up to 30% of course time may be used in contracting and feedback. (To see how contracting is used in group education, see the course protocol in Appendix 3B.)

If education is given on a one-on-one basis, the feedback mechanism should also be institutionalized. This can be done by noting the contract in the chart and asking about it on the next visit. Better yet is a quick phone call in a week to 10 days to see how the contract is going.

Modeling

One of the best ways of helping to enhance efficacy and change behavior is to allow the person changing the behavior to see someone else with the same problem. This is the principle used by the American Cancer Society in its Reach for Recovery program, in which women who have had mastectomies visit new mastectomy patients. It is also one of the reasons that support groups are so popular and successful. In choosing models, one should look for someone who is as much like the patient as possible. Thus matching should be done by age, sex, ethnic origin, and socioeconomic status.

Unfortunately, as health educators, we often use the wrong types of models. For want of a better word, we will call these "superachievers." These are people who have had problems and have overcome them in some spectacular manner. An example would be the marathon runner who lost a leg to cancer, or the older woman with two hip replacements who, after hiking all day, does Scottish dancing. Although these people are real inspirations, they are not the best models. Their achievements, to most of us, just do not seem realistic. A better model is someone who has a problem and is coping with it on a day-to-day basis. This is the type of person to whom your clients can relate.

One might use models in several ways. One way is to use lay instructors with the problem. This is the model used by the Arthritis Self-Help Course. Given a structured curriculum, good training, and adequate professional backup, lay people can make excellent health education instructors. People with problems can also be brought into health education classes to talk with clients and to share experiences. Be careful, when choosing models, not to choose superachievers.

Another way of using models is to have class members help each other. This is done by allowing the class members, rather than the instructor, to solve problems. Every time a problem is stated, the leader should ask the group if anyone has ever had a similar problem or has any ideas about how to solve the problem. The leader should always be the expert of last resort. This teaching strategy has several advantages. First, it teaches class members that they really are experts and have useful knowledge to share. It also teaches them that they do not always have to rely on professionals for expert help. It generates many innovative solutions to problems that would probably never be thought of by professional instructors. Finally, this approach allows patients who most often depend on others to become helpers. This helper role is much valued.

All health education media should demonstrate appropriate modeling. This includes videos, tapes, books, and pamphlets. If the audience is made up largely of South Sea islanders, then the relaxation tape should be recorded by a South

Sea islander. If you are teaching older people how to get up from the floor after falling, then the pictures you use should be of a slightly overweight older person, not a slim, lithe young man or woman. Unfortunately, most health education media choose their models for their physical or charismatic qualities rather than for their ability to act as role models. One note of caution: Be careful when using caricatures or humorous drawings. These may be offensive to some patients. In fact, patients have often told us to limit the "humor" in our written materials. They tell us that disease is not funny.

Reinterpretation of Physiological Signs and Symptoms

For the most part, people who are not mentally or cognitively impaired act rationally. At least, their actions are rational within their own belief system. However, as health professionals, we see many actions that do not seem rational. Our job is to determine why people believe as they do and then, when possible, change these beliefs. This is especially true when it comes to disease symptoms. For example, one of the symptoms common to many chronic conditions is fatigue. Patients are usually told to rest or to balance work with rest. It is only recently that we have come to realize that many people with chronic illness are also depressed. Fatigue is a symptom of depression. However, in the case of depression, resting will only exacerbate the fatigue. Therefore it should be explained to patients that fatigue can come from the disease, in which case resting is a good idea. However, it may also come from depression, in which case exercise may help. Given this explanation, suggest that when people are fatigued, they try exercising. About half the people will find this beneficial and the rest will become more fatigued, in which case they should rest rather than exercise.

Sometimes health professionals give mixed messages. For example, we still sometimes talk about sugar diabetes. Is it then a wonder that patients are confused and think that sugar causes diabetes?

Determining someone's beliefs about a disease is not difficult. All one needs to do is ask. Questions that are helpful in soliciting beliefs are (a) If you _____ (stop smoking, start exercising, etc.), what are you afraid might happen? (b) When you think of_____ (dieting, cancer, etc.), what do you think of? and (c) Why don't you _____?

Once you have identified the belief, you can set out to reinterpret it. Here it is very important to listen to your language. What you say may not be what you mean. In arthritis we talk about "joint protection," which means using joints in an appropriate, nonstressful way. However, some patients interpret this as not using their joints or protecting their marijuana stash. Keeping language simple serves everyone's best interests.

Persuasion

This is the last way of enhancing efficacy and probably the way most familiar to health educators. Persuasion can take many forms, from fear arousal to social support. One aspect of persuasion that seems especially powerful is to use health care providers and patient educators to urge clients toward doing slightly more than they are now doing. Goals should be short-term and realistic. Most important, they should not be much beyond what the clients believe they can *now* accomplish. Thus, instead of saying, "You could lose 20 pounds if you tried," it would be better to say, "You could lose 5 to 6 pounds this month."

In summary, self-efficacy is the belief that one can perform some future behavior or use some cognitive strategy such as stress reduction. It can be enhanced by skills mastery, model-ing, reinterpretation of physiological signs and symptoms, and persuasion.

Stress and Coping Theory

It is a generally accepted concept that one of the major functions of patient education is to help patients cope with the problems caused by changing health habits or illness. However, few patient educators ever look carefully at the coping theory literature. The following discussion focuses on the work of Lazarus and Folkman (1984). It should be emphasized that this is only one of many coping theories and that it was chosen because it fits well with self-efficacy theory and has practical applications in the real world.

Lazarus and Folkman (1984) defined coping as the per-son's constantly changing cognitive and behavioral efforts to manage specific external and/or internal demands that are appraised as taxing or exceeding the person's resources. This definition has several key points. First, coping efforts are not constant over time but rather are ever changing in response to new situations. Obviously, people cope differently given differ-ent situations. For example, one might have little problem in losing weight, yet be unable to stop smoking. Also, the way someone copes today may be very different from the way he or she copes tomorrow, even in similar situations. Second, coping efforts are both behavioral and cognitive. That is, people do things and think in different ways in order to meet specific situations. Third, to stimulate coping efforts, the situation must seem taxing or overwhelming to the individual. The reality of the situation as seen by others has little to do with how a specific person sees the same situation. This is why different people react to the same situation in very different ways. For example, one person may view minor surgery as a relatively unimportant inconvenience, whereas for another person the same surgery can become a major, frightening event. The first person may not need to use any unusual coping strategies, whereas the second may need many strategies in order to cope successfully.

Two kinds of factors influence stress and coping responses: personal factors and situational factors. Personal factors are all those things that the individual brings to the situation—most important, his or her personal life experience and history. Situational factors are just that—situational. Seeing a lion at the zoo probably does not arouse any stress; seeing one on a safari in Africa may arouse some excitement but probably little fear; encountering a hungry mountain lion while hiking on a narrow mountain track may arouse a great deal of anxiety. In all three cases, the stimulus, a lion, is the same. However, the situations are very different. The same is true for patients. A fever in a 3-month-old is quite different from the same fever in a 6-year-old. Thus stress is caused by how the individual sees or appraises both personal and situational factors.

In effect, appraisal is the key to how a person interprets a stressor and how he or she reacts to it. This is similar to our discussion of self-efficacy and how beliefs determine how one reacts to a specific physiological sign or symptom. Appraisal is one's way of evaluating a situation and determining whether a threat exists. There are two types of appraisal: primary and secondary. Primary appraisal is a judgment about whether an event creates a sense of harm or loss. The health belief model discussed later in this chapter would call this "perceived threat." Thus, for someone very concerned with cancer, a breast lump may create a sense of potential harm or loss, whereas for someone ignorant of the warning signs of cancer, a painless breast lump may have no significance. Secondary appraisal is the judgment as to whether the situation is changeable or control-lable. For someone who has seen his or her grandparents live

208PATIENTEDUCATION

full lives as diabetics, diabetes may seem controllable. For another person who has had a friend die from diabetes, the diagnosis of this disease may be a catastrophic event. The difference is that the first person's secondary appraisal is of a controllable event, whereas the second person's is of an uncontrollable event. Secondary appraisal is very much like the expectation step in the health belief model (discussed later in this chapter), in which the individual determines the potential for personal control (Becker, 1974). Self-efficacy can also be considered a way of expressing secondary appraisal.

So far we have examined how someone's appraisal of a situation influences his or her response. Let us now look at the common coping responses used in illness situations. This list of responses is not all-inclusive and may change depending on which researcher created the list. It is presented to give the patient education practitioner some ideas about the types of coping strategies that might be included in a health education program.

Lazarus and Folkman (1984) identified eight distinct ways of coping: confronting, distancing, self-control, seeking social support, accepting responsibility, escape-avoidance, problem solving, and positive reappraisal. We now examine each of these a bit further.

1. *Confronting* is probably not a useful way of dealing with an illness, as there is no way an illness can respond. On the other hand, if the problem is another person's actions in response to the illness, then confronting may be a very useful strategy. For example, if a spouse is nonsupportive, confronting may be a useful coping mechanism. In this instance, an appropriate strategy would be teaching patients to report their own feelings rather than to blame their spouses for lack of support. Confrontative communication can also be used in helping people to take action on destructive behaviors, such as drinking. Thus

"tough love" is a form of confrontational coping (York, York, & Wachtel, 1982).

2. *Distancing* is the strategy by which people separate themselves from the problem. They somehow convince themselves that their condition is different from anyone else's and that therefore they cannot benefit from the experience of others. The person who distances is the one who comes to a class or support group and complains because the people in the group are different from him or her. In some cases, this complaint is realistic. However, in others, it is just a way of saying, "I am coping with my problem by distancing myself from it."

3. *Self-control* is a coping strategy highly encouraged by most health educators. It is taking an active interest in coping with the problem by taking control and practicing such activities as self-care and active decision making. The one caution about self-control is that if it is encouraged too much it may result in victim blaming. For example, someone who has deformities after a stroke should be encouraged to exercise. However, the deformities should never be blamed on that person's lack of exercise. Also, given highly unpredictable or uncontrollable situations, the unfettered use of self-control can lead to learned helplessness (discussed later in this chapter). One thing clients need to learn is the difference between what they can and cannot control. Trying to control the uncontrollable can be very counterproductive.

4. *Seeking social support* is a well-known coping mechanism. Needless to say, it is usually considered a useful and productive coping mechanism. The perception of people's support is probably more important than the amount of support. In other words, one person may have a loving family with a lot of support but perceive that he or she has little support. Another person may have little support from a friend but perceive that he or she has good support. In this case, the second person may cope better than the first. Patient education programs should try to build not only the amount of support but also the patient's perception of the support. A final note: There is a

growing literature that giving support (being helpful to others) may be as important as getting support. Patient education programs should be structured to foster the helper role.

5. *Accepting responsibility* is a coping mechanism that applies more to business than to illness. Although some illnesses may be due to one's past actions, trying to get someone to accept responsibility is probably counterproductive and only adds to victim blaming. On the other hand, taking personal responsibility is extremely important for preventive practices. Thus this coping strategy is most useful when used selectively.

6. *Escape-avoidance*, like other strategies, can be either good or bad. Sometimes, the best thing to do with a problem is not to deal with it. However, in the case of most illnesses, this is not possible. Avoidance may be a good short-term solution but usually does not work in the long run.

7. *Problem solving* is one of the most useful strategies for coping with illness. Unfortunately, most patient education programs teach solutions, not the problem-solving process. It is like feeding the starving man a fish instead of teaching him how to fish. Problem solving, therefore, is a coping strategy that should be more utilized (D'Zurilla, 1986).

8. *Positive reappraisal* is a strategy used successfully by many people with illness. Instead of dwelling on what they cannot do, they work at being successful at what they can do. By looking at an illness as a challenge or opportunity, many people have been able to accomplish things that they would have never done if not faced with the illness. Again, this is a strategy that deserves emphasis in health education programs.

Rosenstiel and Keefe (1983) identified the coping strategies used by patients with low back pain as reinterpreting, activity, distraction, self-talk, ignoring, and prayer. Two of these strategies, reinterpreting and ignoring, are old friends: Lazarus and Folkman (1984) called them positive reappraisal and escape-avoidance. Let us now examine the others.

1. *Activity* is fairly self-explanatory. Activity is an excellent coping strategy, especially when dealing with pain or depression or trying to change habits such as eating or smoking. This strategy can cover many things, including physical activity, such as walking or swimming, and more passive activities, such as knitting, reading, or painting. Generally, doing something is better than doing nothing.

2. *Distraction* is a coping strategy for pain, depression, and changing of habits. It works on the principle that the human mind, like a radio, cannot be tuned into two things at the same time. Therefore, if the mind is occupied, pain, depression, and other cognitive problems are lessened. Distraction can take many forms, including going to see a funny movie or counting backwards from 100 by threes to help insomnia. The principle is that, whatever the activity, the mind must be kept fully occupied. In recent years, humor has been used as such a coping mechanism. This is just one of many forms of distraction.

3. *Self-talk* is a variation on positive thinking. All of us talk to ourselves all the time: for example, "I don't really want to get up, it is too cold." Self-talk can be either a negative or a positive coping strategy because it often becomes a self-fulfilling prophecy. In helping clients use self-talk constructively, have them write down the conversations they have with themselves and then change all the negative talk to positive talk: for example, "I don't really want to get up, but if I do I can read the paper and have a cup of tea."

4. *Prayer* is one coping strategy that is often ignored by health educators. Somehow we feel that this is best left to the individual or to the clergy. However, for certain segments of the population, it is a very powerful and useful mechanism that should be used more often. One innovative use of prayer and religion was exemplified by a U.S. arthritis program serving a rural southern population. Many of the justifications for self-help activities were backed with biblical quotes. Also, if people had a problem with the

relaxation exercises, they were instructed to substitute silent prayer.

In conclusion, stress and coping theory provides us with many ideas for use in patient education. Patient educators should take the time and effort to formalize the teaching of coping strategies in their programs. Not all strategies will work for all patients. However, if a variety are offered, the chances are greater that individuals will find something of value.

Learned-Helplessness Theory

Learned helplessness is a third theory drawn from social psychology that is relevant to healthful behavior change. The theory evolved from the animal research of Seligman and Maier (1967). They observed that dogs that had learned that shock was inescapable, no matter how they responded, became unresponsive or helpless. In social psychological terms, the dogs learned that shock was "noncontingent," that it occurred independently of their actions. No matter what they did, they were shocked! A sense of "noncontingency," the recognition that an event such as shock occurs independently of one's actions, is the basic cause of learned helplessness.

This initial conceptualization led to much discussion about the relevance of learned helplessness to human behavior, controversy about the causes of helplessness, and eventually the development and elaboration of the learned-helplessness model by Seligman (1975). The theory is primarily an attempt to understand or explain how a sense of noncontingency develops. Three causes or "causal attributions" were identified: (a) internal versus external, (b) global versus specific, and (c) stable versus unstable. These three attributions are related, but we will look first at each separately.

The first dimension distinguishes between universal and personal helplessness. This dimension describes a continuum of attributional style referred to as *internality versus externality*. The frame of reference used to determine an individual's relative placement on this continuum is the familiar self-other dichotomy. Simply stated, an individual may believe that noncontingency between response and outcome can be attributed solely to internal, personal factors. An individual at the opposite end of the continuum may attribute noncontingency to external, universal factors.

For example, a smoker who attributes failure to stop smoking to lack of will power is operating in a personal helplessness mode. He or she may believe that lack of will power is a fatal flaw and that failure is inevitable, and thus give up trying. Another smoker may ascribe a similar problem to social pressure or genes. This person is considered to be operating in a universal helplessness mode, emphasizing external causes that may or may not be remediable.

The second dimension distinguishes between global and specific helplessness. *Global helplessness* means that learned-helplessness deficits occur across a wide range of situations, from driving a car to holding a job to losing weight. *Specific helplessness* means that the deficits occur across a narrow range of situations. For example, a person could drive a car and hold a job but be totally unsuccessful at losing weight. Attributing failure to global factors results in helplessness generalizable to other situations ("I cannot drive a car, hold a job, or lose weight"). When attributed to specific factors, however, helplessness deficits occur only in the original situation ("I cannot lose weight").

The third dimension involves the influence of learned-helplessness deficits occurring occasionally or consistently over time. This dimension consists of a continuum of stable to unstable attributions. *Stable attributions* are generally recurrent factors; *unstable attributions* are short-lived or intermittent factors. For example, one might never be able to lose weight, a stable attribution, or one might be unable to lose weight only during the Christmas holidays, an unstable attribution. Psychologists also call this a *trait-state distinction:* Traits are stable attributes; states are transitory.

The descriptions of attributional style are interrelated. Internal attributions are apt to be more stable and global than external attributions. These links are not, however, invariant and should never be assumed. Thus an individual's relative placement on *each* of the three continua in a *particular* situation determines his or her helplessness deficit. It also assists to some extent in predicting the occurrence of future deficits.

These causal attributions lead to an expectation of failure or lack of control, which, in turn, results in the deficits termed *learned helplessness*—that is, deficits in motivation, cognition, and action. Problem-solving attempts occur infrequently: For example, the typical response is "What difference does it make?" Depression is a common result of learned helplessness.

Comparison With Other Theories

Learned-helplessness theory encompasses some of the same concerns as self-efficacy and stress and coping theories. For example, learned helplessness includes behaviors as well as thoughts and feelings, self-efficacy focuses on behaviors, and stress and coping considers thoughts, feelings, and behaviors. The learned-helplessness model does not, however, *directly* suggest either appropriate coping behaviors or theory-derived intervention, as do self-efficacy and stress and coping theories. On the other hand, it may better explain human responses to some diseases in which there is often a notable lack of relationship between most behaviors and resulting clinical outcomes

(Lorig & Laurin, 1985). Multiple sclerosis is well known for its unpredictable, even capricious "flares" or exacerbations and remissions, particularly in its physical manifestations. Unpredictability and capriciousness are close in meaning to, if not synonymous with, noncontingency. This suggests that intervention may need to emphasize cognitive and emotional ways of handling uncertainty.

Theory-Based Practice Guidelines

Interventions that may be effective in lessening learned helplessness include strategies similar to those mentioned earlier and are derived from self-efficacy and stress and coping theories: skills mastery, modeling, reinterpreting or cognitive restructuring of the signs and symptoms of disease, and problem- and emotion-focused ways of coping. Cognitive restructuring may be one of the most important, so it will be reexamined briefly. It is an important approach to increasing clients' beliefs in personal control of their interpersonal and social environments.

The critical factor in determining an individual's response is not the actual situation as much as how the person labels or evaluates the situation. This is also the basis of the health belief model (discussed later in this chapter). If negative emotions are roused because individuals unthinkingly accept certain illogical premises or irrational ideas, then teaching clients to think more logically and rationally may create positive emotional states that change behavior in healthful directions. It is, for example, more rational to believe "I have difficulty losing weight" than "I'll never be thin." "Difficulties" can be managed; if one can "never" be thin, change will be unsuccessful.

The specific steps of intervention using cognitive restructuring are as follows:

1. *Helping clients accept the fact that self-statements mediate emotions.* The self-statement "I'll never be thin" arouses helplessness, whereas the statement "I have difficulty in losing weight" represents a challenge (see discussion of self-talk earlier in this chapter).

2. *Assisting clients to recognize the irrationality of certain beliefs.* The patient educator should ask the client to consider the following questions: What evidence supports my belief? Which parts of my beliefs are true, and which parts are false? Am I distorting events? That is, what data suggest that I will *never* lose weight? Can I lose weight but still not be "thin"? Is "thinness" a realistic goal?

3. *Helping clients understand that the inability to initiate or sustain desirable behaviors frequently results from irrational self-statements.* Negative emotional responses can be maintained easily and indefinitely by irrational thinking. Clients need, among other things, to stop thinking irrationally in order to facilitate constructive behavior changes.

4. *Helping clients modify their irrational self-statements.* Have the client write down rational self-statements and rehearse them in role-playing situations. Imaginary presentations of troublesome situations—a colleague's going-away party replete with pastries and junk food, for example—can be described to the client by the patient educator, and rational self-statements can be practiced.

In summary, learned helplessness occurs most frequently in situations in which the client believes he or she has little control. The result of helplessness is often depression. Learned helplessness can be overcome by reconstructing thoughts and self-statements.

¤ TWO MODELS: *PRECEDE* AND THE HEALTH BELIEF MODEL

In planning a patient education program, it is necessary to have a rationale and one or more theories. Then you can use a model to put these all together. A model is a planning tool that gives you the outline with which to continue. We describe two models: PRECEDE and the health belief model (Green, Kruter, 1991; Becker, 1974; Rosentock, 1990). Both have been widely used in health promotion and patient education programs. Again, like theory, there is no one perfect model. Rather, you will have to choose the one that best meets your needs.

The PRECEDE Model

The PRECEDE model (*P*receding, *R*einforcing, *E*nabling *C*auses in *E*ducational *D*iagnosis and *E*valuation) suggests looking at three factors when planning a patient education program: predisposing, enabling, and reinforcing factors.

Predisposing Factors

Predisposing factors can largely be divided into two categories—beliefs and benefits. Your job is to discover what these are. People generally act in a rational manner—at least, they have reasons for doing what they do, although you may not agree with them. However, there are always reasons. For example, if someone believes that exercise will cause a second heart attack, it is not surprising that he or she does not want to exercise. In the same vein, if someone thinks that taking a medication will have serious side effects, it is no wonder that he or she does not take the medication.

In order to change beliefs, you must first find out what they are. You can usually do this by asking one of the following questions: "What are you afraid might happen if you _____?" (Fill in the blank with the desired behavior, such as "take medication" or "exercise"); "Why don't you _____?" (Fill in a health behavior); or "What do you think causes _____?" (Fill in the blank with a symptom such as pain).

Once you know a belief, you can set out to change it. You can usually do this through explanation—for example:

> I can understand why you might think that muscle-relaxing exercises would not help pain. However, when you have pain, the muscles in the area become tense. These tense muscles can cause more pain. You can help this in two ways: (a) by strengthening the muscles with appropriate exercise, and (b) by learning how to relax the muscles with muscle relaxation techniques. Would you like me to show you how to strengthen and relax your muscles?

Sometimes you cannot change a belief. If this belief is very important to the individual or is widely held in the culture, it may be very hard to change. In such cases, you may not have to change the belief, especially if it is not interfering with behavior change. Rather, you can add to an existing belief—for example:

> I know that you believe that God cures everything and that prayer is very important. I agree. In biblical times, Sophocles said, "Heaven ne'er helps the man who will not act." This was later translated by the American Ben Franklin to "God helps them that help themselves." Don't you think that your prayers might work better if you gave God a little help?

In both these cases, helping someone change or add to his or her beliefs would be helpful in accomplishing both behavior change and enhancing self-efficacy.

Another predisposing factor that can get in the way of behavior change is secondary gain that can come from having an illness. People may use illness as a reason for not working, as a way of getting the family to do chores, or as a way of getting attention and sympathy from friends. If this is the case, one has very little motivation for getting better and many reasons for not changing behaviors. No behavior change will take place until the benefits are changed. If family and friends ignore illness behaviors but give encouragement to new healthful behaviors, the reward structure changes. This is sometimes a very delicate matter. You must plan a program that includes family members and then work with the whole family to change the benefits.

As a patient educator, you may actually contribute to the problem. For example, some people in patient education classes always have an excuse for not doing something. We sometimes call them "Yes, But" people. By their actions, they force you and other class members to spend a lot of time with them. In this case, it is best to cut them short and spend your time with people you can help (this is discussed more in Chapter 7).

A third set of predisposing factors has to do with lack of resources. People may not take part in education or healthful behaviors because they lack time or fiscal resources. In this case, your job is to help them understand how they can make the behavior change given their life circumstances and schedule your educational activities at times and places that make attendance possible (see Chapter 5).

Enabling Factors

These are the factors that help people do something they really believe they should do and want to do but are not able to do because things such as the complexity of the regime, distance, lack of skills, or lack of ability get in the way. There are two major ways to enable people: finding resources and skills mastery. In both these cases, the major objective is to assist the person in gaining control. This is important to keep in mind, for many times people will try to get you to do something that they could well do themselves. For example, do not get trapped into always providing transportation. See if someone else in the class or a family member can do this. Usually, if patients want to do something bad enough, they will find a way. By always supplying easy answers, you are keeping the person dependent. Sometimes being too helpful can be harmful.

Try not to solve problems but rather to teach problem-solving skills. Work with the individual to find what is needed. Brainstorm ideas about where one might find resources, make suggestions about resources, or even look up resources if necessary. Then plan with the individual how he or she will make contact with the resource and how it will be used. In other words, supply information but not direct help unless it is absolutely necessary.

Reinforcing Factors

Once people have decided to do something, whether they continue doing it is largely dependent on reinforcing factors. These include the support of family and friends, the opinions of their doctor and other health care providers, and their satisfaction or dissatisfaction with the results. Again, you can do a great deal to assist with the reinforcement. This includes arranging for the use of modeling and persuasion (discussed earlier in this chapter).

Another important way of reinforcing behavior change is through inclusion of family, friends, and health providers in your educational efforts. If the family is supportive and not nagging, and the providers are interested in the behavior changes and encouraging, this can make all the difference. Do

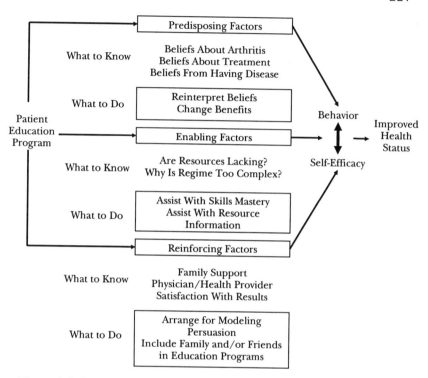

Figure 9.3. Integration of PRECEDE Model and Self-Efficacy Theory

not leave these important components out of your program planning efforts.

Fortunately, we have one final important reinforcing factor. When patients become a bit more confident and start taking their medication, exercising, or otherwise changing to more healthful behaviors, they feel better. This, in turn, reinforces them to continue doing what they are doing.

In conclusion, when planning and implementing the PRECEDE model, examine the predisposing, enabling, and reinforcing factors. Then, using theory, intervene on these as appropriate. Figure 9.3 is an example of how the PRECEDE model and one theory, self-efficacy, might be integrated.

In conclusion, use the PRECEDE model in planning your intervention. Pay close attention to the predisposing, enabling, and reinforcing factors that either help or impede behavior change. Then use theory to form an intervention that will influence the most important factors.

Health Belief Model

The health belief model is one of the oldest and most widely used health education models. It was originally formulated during the 1950s (Becker, 1974) to explain why people did not go for tuberculosis screening. Since that time, it has undergone revision and has been used to plan many programs. The basis of this model is that people act on the basis of perceptions. These can be divided into two major classes: perceived threat and expectations. Let us examine these more closely.

Perceived Threat

If someone does not see something as threatening, then there is no reason to act. There are two levels of perceived threat: perceived susceptibility and perceived severity. Most people perceive AIDS as a severe disease. However, there are many different beliefs about susceptibility. Safe sex will be practiced only by those who believe themselves to be susceptible. On the other hand, one might believe that one is susceptible to getting the flu but still get on the bus with someone who has the flu. In this case, the individual is less concerned with severity.

To change health behaviors, one usually must believe in both susceptibility and severity. This is one reason that many people "get religion" after they have been diagnosed with cancer or heart disease. At this point, they believe themselves susceptible and thus finally give up smoking or lose weight.

Expectations

Beliefs in severity and susceptibility are not enough. People must also have the expectations that (a) the new behavior will be beneficial, (b) the barriers to change do not outweigh the benefits, and (c) they can accomplish the needed behavior change (our old friend, self-efficacy, discussed earlier in this chapter).

This is like a cost-benefit analysis. Many people do not like taking arthritis or hypertension medications because of side effects. In the case of arthritis, they would rather have painful joints then gastrointestinal problems. With hypertension, the problem is more complex because there are usually no symptoms. Therefore, unless one has a strong belief in severity and susceptibility, the barriers—side effects—can easily outweigh the benefits.

Unfortunately, for many behaviors, the barriers are immediate and the benefits long-range. Said another way, the barriers are certain unpleasantness that needs to be weighed against not-so-certain future benefits. An example is not eating chocolate cake now in the hopes of not having cancer or a stroke in the future. From this perspective, it is not hard to see why it is so difficult to get patients to change behaviors. On the other hand, a patient, by definition, already has a problem. Thus the cost-benefit ratio is more in favor of behavior change.

Two more aspects of the health belief model should be mentioned. To a great extent, one's expectations are shaped by background factors (the PRECEDE model would call these predisposing factors; see discussion earlier in this chapter). Also, cues to action seem to have an important role in deter-

mining if one actually changes behavior. For example, someone may know that being overweight is unhealthy and that
dieting will reduce weight. She might also feel she has the skills
to lose weight but still nothing happens. During a routine
checkup, our mythical person finds she has high systolic blood
pressure. This cue moves her to a weight control program. Cues
are elusive; they really cannot be planned. However, by providing patients with examples and with hints on how to get started
easily, we can hope to supply the necessary cue. Of course,
some cues are external and hit hard, such as a stroke or the
death of a friend from cancer.

¤ CONCLUSION

In this chapter we have examined a rationale, three theories, and two models that are useful in planning patient education programs. The purpose in providing this material is to give
you some tools with which to build a program. Putting together
a good patient education program is a little like building a
house. You need a grand design. This is provided by the models
and theories you choose to incorporate. Will your house be
made of bricks, wood, or concrete? Will it have two bedrooms
or five? If you do not have a plan in mind, you will probably get
a mess. Next, you need the materials—the actual bricks, wood,
glass, nails, and so forth. This is the content of your course,
what you are going to teach. Much of this content was determined in your needs assessment. Finally, you need tools. These
help you put your materials together in an efficient manner
that turns the raw material into the home of your dreams. In
patient education, the tools are the processes through which
you choose to deliver your content. These processes are discussed in Chapter 3. Just as you would not build a house using

just one tool, no matter how useful, you should not build a patient education program using just one process. As a patient educator, you are the contractor. The final design and product are up to you.

¤ NOTE

1. *Patient Education and Counseling* is published quarterly. For subscription information, write Elsevier Scientific Publishers, Customer Relations Manager, Ireland Ltd., Bay 15, Shannon Industrial Estate, County Clare, Ireland. *Health Education Quarterly* is published by Sage Publications. For subscription information, write Sage Publications, Inc., 2455 Teller Road, Thousand Oaks, CA 91320.

¤ BIBLIOGRAPHY

Bandura, A. (1982). Self-efficacy in human agency. *American Psychologist, 37,* 122-147.

Bandura, A. (1986). *Social foundations of thoughts and action.* Englewood Cliffs, NJ: Prentice Hall.

Bandura, A. (1991). Self-efficacy mechanism in psychological activation and health promoting behavior. In J. Madden, IV (Ed.), *Neurobiology of learning, emotion, and affect* (pp. 229-268). New York: Raven Press Ltd.

Becker, M. (Ed.). (1974). The health belief model and personal health behavior. *Health Education Monographs, 2,* 236.

D'Zurilla, T. J. (1986). *Problem solving therapy.* New York: Springer.

Lazarus, R. S., & Folkman, S. (1984). *Stress appraisal and coping.* New York: Springer.

Fries, J. F., & Crapo, L. M. (1981). *Vitality and aging.* San Francisco: W. H. Freeman.

Glanz, R., Rimer, B., & Lewis, F. (Eds.). (1990). *Health behavior and health education: Theory, research, and practice.* San Francisco: Jossey-Bass.

Green, L. W., & Kruter, M. W. (1991). *Health promotion planning: An educational and environmental approach.* Mountain View, CA: Mayfield.

Houland, C. I. (Ed.). (1957). *The order of presentation in persuasion.* New Haven, CT: Yale University Press.

Lorig, K., & Laurin, J. (1985). Some notions about assumptions underlying health education. *Health Education Quarterly, 12,* 231-243.

Rosenstiel, A. R., & Keefe, F. J. (1983). The use of coping strategies in chronic low back pain patients: Relationship to patient characteristics and current adjustment. *Pain, 17,* 33-40.

Rosentock, I. M. (1990). The health belief model: Explaining health behavior through expectancies. In R. Glanz, B. Rimer, & F. Lewis (Eds.), *Health behavior and health education: Theory, research, and practice* (pp. 39-62). San Francisco: Jossey-Bass.

Schwarzer, R. (1992). *Self-efficacy: Thought control of action.* Philadelphia: Hemisphere.

Seligman, M. (1975). *Helplessness: On depression, development, and death.* San Francisco: W. H. Freeman.

Seligman, M., & Maier, S. (1967). Failure to escape traumatic shock. *Journal of Experimental Psychology, 74,* 1-9.

Wallston, B. S., Wallston, K. A., Kaplan, G. D., & Maides, S. A. (1976). Development and validation of the health locus of control (HLC) scale. *Journal of Consulting and Clinical Psychology, 44,* 580-585.

York, P., York, D., & Wachtel, T. (1982). *Tough love.* New York: Bantam.

10

Joint Commission on Accreditation of Healthcare Organizations (JCAHO)
Patient and Family Education Regulations

Mary M. Hobbs

If you work in a hospital, or a clinic attached to a hospital, you are required to design and document your patient teaching to

The regulations quoted in this chapter are from the *1995 Comprehensive Accreditation Manual for Hospitals.* Oakbrook Terrace, IL: Joint Commission on Accreditation of Healthcare Organizations, 1994, pp. 189-205. Reprinted with permission.

meet Joint Commission on Accreditation of Healthcare Organizations (JCAHO) regulations regarding patient and family education (JCAHO, 1994). These first appeared in the *1993 Accreditation Manual for Hospitals* and were further consolidated and defined in the 1994 manual. In the 1994 manual, the chapter on patient and family education contains the requirements that were previously contained in the chapters on dietetic services, hospital-sponsored ambulatory care services, medical record services, nursing care, patient rehabilitation services, special care units, and surgical and anesthesia services.

Much of the information in this book is helpful in meeting these guidelines. Although many of the references in this book refer to group teaching, you will find that you can readily apply the principles to one-on-one teaching.

Figure 10.1 is a sample Multidisciplinary Patient Education Form that can be used to document inpatient education and referrals to outpatient education or other educational resources. This form is a composite of forms from several hospitals. Please note that it has not been used in a JCAHO accreditation visit. It was developed because JCAHO surveyors have been expressing their preference for *one* documentation form in the inpatient record, on which every educational intervention is noted. This single form is designed for use by nurses, respiratory therapists, dietitians, physical therapists, and so forth. If more detailed notes are required, the form refers to the section in the chart where that note can be found.

Listed in this chapter are the 1994 JCAHO Patient and Family Education regulations, followed by references to the sections in this book that will assist you in meeting those requirements. Readers should note that there may be more recent standards as this book was written in mid-1994. If so, these guidelines should still be helpful.

Name:_____

Diagnosis:_____

Learner: ☐ Patient   ☐ Domestic Partner   ☐ Other _____

Initial Learning Assessment
Cultural_____ Desire to learn_____
Religious_____ Hearing_____
Age_____ Sight_____
Language_____ Translator_____
Emotional state_____
Cognitive limitations_____
Physical limitations_____
Other_____

TEACHING CODES	LEARNING CODES
A. Questions answered. B. Verbal information provided. C. Written information provided. D. Task demonstrated. E. Audio/visual used.	1. Needs further instruction. 2. Demonstrates verbal understanding. 3. Return demonstration, with help. 4. Return demonstration, independent.

SUBJECT	TEACH CODE	LEARN CODE	COMMENTS/ SEE ALSO	DATE/ TIME	TEACHER'S INITIAL
Signature/Title		Signature/Title			
Signature/Title		Signature/Title			
Signature/Title		Signature/Title			

Figure 10.1. Sample Multidisciplinary Patient Education Form

NOTE: This form meets the intent of JCAHO. It has not been reviewed at a Joint Commission visit.

PF.1 The patient and/or, when appropriate, his or her family are provided with appropriate education and training to increase knowledge of the patient's illness and treatment needs and to learn skills and behaviors that promote recovery and improve function.

PF.2 The patient and/or, when appropriate, his or her family receive education specific to the patient's assessed needs (a), abilities (b), and readiness (c), and appropriate to the patient's length of stay.

(a) Assessing needs:
Chapter 1. *See especially* "Structured and Semistructured Interviews."
Chapter 3. *See especially* "Setting Priorities: Choosing What to Teach in the Time Allotted."

(b) Assessing abilities:
Chapter 8.

PF.2.1 The patient and/or, when appropriate, his or her family have their learning needs, abilities, and readiness to learn assessed. (See references a and b, PF.1 and PF.2.)

PF.2.1.1 When indicated, the assessment includes cultural and religious practices (a), emotional barriers (b), desire and motivation to learn (c), physical and/or cognitive limitations (d), and language barriers (e).

(a) Assessing cultural and religious practices, and language barriers:
Chapter 6. *See especially* "Understanding Cultural Diversity"; Table 6.1; and "Strategies for Adapting Program Content and Process, subsection "Dispelling Health Misconceptions or Myths."

(b) Assessing desire and motivation to learn and physical and/or cognitive limitations:

Chapter 1. *See especially* "Structured and Semistructured Interviews."

Chapter 3. *See especially* "Setting Priorities: Choosing What to Teach in the Time Allotted."

(c) Physical and/or cognitive limitations:

Chapter 8.

> PF.2.2 The patient and/or, when appropriate, his or her family are provided with the specific knowledge and/or skills required to meet the patient's ongoing health care needs (a). Such instruction is presented in ways understandable to the patient and/or his or her family (b) and includes, but is not limited to,
>
> PF.2.2.1 the safe and effective use of medication in accordance with legal requirements and patient needs, when applicable;
>
> PF.2.2.2 the safe and effective use of medical equipment, when applicable;
>
> PF.2.2.3 instruction and potential drug-food interactions and counseling on nutrition intervention and/or modified diets, as appropriate;
>
> PF.2.2.4 instruction in rehabilitation techniques to facilitate adaptation to and/or functional independence in the environment, if needed;
>
> PF.2.2.5 access to available community resources, if needed;
>
> PF.2.2.6 when and how to obtain further treatment, if needed.

(a) Provided with the knowledge/skills:

Chapter 3. *See especially* "Setting Priorities: Choosing What to Teach in the Time Allotted," "Knowing What and When to Teach," "Knowing How to Teach," "Putting It All Together," "Documenting What You Teach," and Appendix 3B, box "How to Help Someone Make a Contract."

Chapter 7. *See especially* "Strong, Silent Types," "Antagonistic or Belligerent Participants," and "Yes, Buts."

Chapter 8.

Chapter 9. *See especially* "Three Theories," subsection "Self-Efficacy Theory," sub-subsection "Skills Mastery."

(b) Understandable to the patient/family:

Chapter 4.

Chapter 3. *See especially* "Process," subsections "Group Processes" and "Questioning."

Chapter 6. *See especially* "Understanding Cultural Diversity"; Table 6.1; and "Strategies for Adapting Program Content and Process," subsection "Dispelling Health Misconceptions or Myths."

Chapter 8. *See especially* Question 4.

> PF.2.2.7 The patient and/or, when appropriate, his or her family are provided with the specific knowledge and/or skills required to meet the patient's ongoing health care needs. Such instruction is presented in ways understandable to the patient and/or his or her family and includes, but is not limited to, the patient's and family's responsibilities in the patient's care.

This section emphasizes the patient/family responsibility to provide accurate information to their health care providers, to be considerate of other patients, and to comply with instructions. All of the other sections of the book cited above apply here, but especially, Chapter 8.

PF.3 Any discharge instructions given to the patient and/or, when appropriate, his or her family are provided to the organization or individual responsible for the patient's continuing care.

This section requires that the patient, family, or organization responsible for the patient's post-discharge care are clear about the discharge instructions for ongoing care of the patient.

Chapter 3. *See especially* "Knowing What and When to Teach"; "Knowing How to Teach"; "Putting It All Together"; "Process," subsections "Group Processes" and "Questioning"; "Documenting What You Teach"; and Appendix 3B, box "How to Help Someone Make a Contract."

Chapter 8. *See especially* Question 4.

Chapter 9. *See especially* "Three Theories," subsection "Self-Efficacy Theory," sub-subsection "Skills Mastery."

PF.4 The organization plans and supports the provision and coordination of patient and/or, when appropriate, family education activities and resources.

PF.4.1 The organization identifies and provides the educational resources required to achieve its educational objectives.

PF.4.2 The patient and/or, when appropriate, family educational process is interdisciplinary, as appropriate to the care plan.

These requirements address continuity of education across care settings and over a person's life span and include appropriate referrals to community resources. Appropriate educational materials and resources must be available. Staff must be trained as patient educators, and the education provided must be understandable to the patient/family.

(a) Educational resources:

Chapter 3. *See especially* "Setting Priorities: Choosing What to Teach in the Time Allotted," "Knowing What and When to Teach," "Knowing How to Teach," and "Putting It All Together."

Chapter 8.

(b) Understandable to the patient/family:

Chapter 4.

Chapter 3. *See especially* "Process," subsections "Group Processes" and "Questioning."

Chapter 6. *See especially* "Understanding Cultural Diversity"; Table 6.1; and "Strategies for Adapting Program Content and Process," subsection "Dispelling Health Misconceptions or Myths."

Chapter 8. *See especially* Question 4.

¤ BIBLIOGRAPHY

Joint Commission on Accreditation of Healthcare Organizations. (1994). *1995 Comprehensive Accreditation Manual for Hospitals.* Oakbrook Terrace, IL: Author.

Glossary

Acculturation The process by which one acquires the values, practices, and language of another culture.

Adherence. *See* **Compliance**

Assimilation The extreme form of acculturation, in which one loses the cultural practices of origin and completely acquires and adopts a new culture.

Back-translation A method of translation that uses two independent translators. The first translator translates the material from the original language to the new language; the second translator takes the translated material and translates it back into the original language. The two original language versions are then compared to judge the accuracy and appropriateness of the translation.

Balanced incomplete block design A technique for quantifying and prioritizing qualitative data.

Brainstorm A technique by which a group generates as many ideas as possible without placing comment or value on the ideas generated.

Comparison group Subjects chosen to be compared with the treatment subjects in a nonrandom manner.

Compliance (adherence) Following directions.

Cultural diversity The result of interactions between different cultures.

Cultural identity The culture or cultures with which one identifies at any specific time.

Culture Shared set of beliefs, assumptions, values, and practices.

Educational needs assessment Determining in a planned manner the perceived needs of patients, significant others, and/or providers concerning health.

Epi Info A user-friendly, inexpensive data management and statistical analysis software package.

Focus group A group interviewed to obtain information on specific ideas or concerns.

Formative evaluation. *See* **Process evaluation**

Hard-to-reach people People or patients you have problems reaching due to environmental, cultural, or other mediating factors.

Health behavior Any action one takes to maintain or improve health, to prevent disease, or to slow physical or emotional decline.

Health care utilization The frequency with which one uses health care providers or institutions—for example, days in hospital, number of outpatient visits to a physician, or number of home care visits.

Health status One's current physical or emotional functioning. Usually measured in terms of pain, disability, depression, shortness of breath, fatigue, and so on; can also be measured by self-rated overall health.

Measurement instrument. *See* **Scale**

Model Plan or way of organizing things.

Objective data Data that are unbiased; often data that can be verified against another source.

Operational definition Definition of a term for any specific study or context. For example, see **Patient education** for the operational definition of this term as it is used in this book.

Outcome evaluation (also sometimes known as a summative evaluation) An evaluation of how well the objectives of the program were met. Outcomes are usually measured in terms of health behaviors, health status, and/or health care utilization.

Patient A person who has a defined and present health problem.

Patient education A set of planned, educational activities designed to improve patients' health behaviors and/or health status.

Process evaluation (also known as formative evaluation) An evaluation of what goes on during and sometimes before a health education intervention—for example, how many people came, or if the intervention was delivered as written.

Qualitative data Data that are usually in text form, usually descriptive.

Quantitative data Data that are usually in numeric form; data that can be manipulated statistically.

Questionnaire If the questionnaire is measuring only one construct—for example, pain—then it is the same as a scale or a measurement instrument. Sometimes a questionnaire is composed of many scales.

Randomized To assign to one group or another (usually treatment and control) in no particular order and with no specific purpose.

Rationale Statement of reasons.

Reading level The grade level at which individuals read. Adults may be able to read well above their tested "reading level" if the information is important to them.

Rehearsal Practicing of what to say or how to act in a potentially problematic situation before it occurs.

Role play Acting out a situation or interaction in a safe environment.

Salient beliefs The most important beliefs one holds about any given subject.

Scale (also known as measurement instrument) A collection of items or questions used to find out something specific that is not directly observable.

Self-management Being responsible for and making decisions about one's health. This includes monitoring one's health, making informed decisions about when to use health care providers, practicing appropriate health behaviors, using a problem-solving approach to make decisions, and using family, friends, and community resources as appropriate and necessary.

Self-monitoring Keeping track of one's symptoms or behaviors. The information from self-monitoring is often used to make decisions about medications and/or health behaviors.

Sensitivity This is the degree to which a scale or instrument responds to change. If it responds only to large changes, it is not very sensitive. If it responds to small changes, it is sensitive.

Subjective data Data coming from one's mind; often cannot be verified against another source.

Summative evaluation. *See* **Outcome evaluation**

Theory System of ideas used to explain a particular phenomenon.

Valid Something is valid if it measures truthfully what the evaluator wants to measure.

Index

Accreditation, 95
  JCAHO guidelines, 227-234
Acculturation, 153, 155
Activity, as coping strategy, 211
Advertising, 141, 144-145. *See also*
  Marketing and promotion
Advocacy role, 164
Aging-associated morbidity, 197
AIDS misconceptions, 162
Antagonistic patients, 178
Art, 165
Arthritis self-help course, 100-115,
  203
Assimilation, 153
Asthma, 85, 118
Attention-seeking patients, 173
Attributional style, 212-214
Audiovisual media, 78. *See also*
  Materials; Media
Avoidance, 210

Back-translation, 168-169
Balanced incomplete block design,
  12-16

Bandura, A., 193, 199
Behavioral change:
  compliance, 183-193
  cross-cultural issues, 162-164
  enabling factors, 219-220
  expectations, 223
  models, 202-204
  perceived threat and, 222
  predisposing factors, 217-219
  reinforcing factors, 220-221
  self-efficacy changes and, 201
  target behaviors, 68-70
Beliefs. *See* Patient beliefs
Block design, 12-16
Blood pressure monitoring, 84
Brainstorming, 10, 78-80, 174, 186
Breast self-examination, 87-88

Capability perceptions, 192-193. *See
  also* Self-efficacy
Causal attributions, 212
Center for Epidemiologic Studies
  Depression Scale (CES-D),
  58-60

Charting, 95-96
Choices, 94
Cholesterol, 69
Cloze readability formula, 122
Clubs, 147
Coaching, 80-81
Coding, 36
Cognitive restructuring, 215-216
Community resources, 146-149
Comparison group, 43-44
Compliance, 183-193
   patient understanding and, 188
   self-efficacy beliefs, 192-193
   Self-Reported Medication
     Taking Scale, 61
Comprehensibility, 119, 121-128
   compliance and, 188
   JCAHO guidelines, 232, 234
Computer-based education (CBE),
   77
Computer tools, 17
Confidentiality, 136
Confronting, 208
Consumer Satisfaction Survey, 62-65
Contracting, 111-114, 202
Control, 31
Control (comparison) groups,
   43-44
Coping theory, 206-212
Cost, 138-140
Cost-benefit analysis, 223
Crapo, L. M., 197
Cultural issues, 151-154
   adapting content and process,
     160-166
   creating appropriate programs,
     158-160
   ethnicity, 154-155
   identifying target cultures,
     154-156
   information sources, 156-158
   JCAHO guidelines, 230
   program tips, 164-166

translations, 166-170
Culture, 152

Dance, 165
Data analysis tool, 17
Data collection and analysis, 35-42
Delphi process, 8
Depression, 204
Depression Scale, 58-60
Diabetic self-monitoring, 84, 120
Diet, 69, 83, 159, 163
Disability Index, Health Assessment
   Questionnaire, 49-57
Distancing, 209
Distraction, 211
Diversity. See Cultural issues
Doctors:
   educational role of, 87-88
   marketing programs to, 132-136
Documentation, 95-96
   JCAHO guidelines, 227-228
Drama, 165

Educational materials. See Materials
Efficacy. See Self-efficacy
Epi Info, 17, 38
Escape-avoidance, 210
Ethnicity, 154-155. See also Cultural
   issues
Evaluation, 19-44
   asking the right questions,
     25-26, 30-35
   data collection and analysis,
     35-42
   methods, 26-30
   scales, 32-34, 46-65
   study design, 42-44
   terminology, 20-24
Exercise, 83-84, 148, 183-184
Expectations, 223
Externality, 213

Factor analysis, 33
Family involvement, 165, 191, 220
Fatigue symptoms, 204
Feedback, 192, 202
Fees and costs, 138-140
Field testing, 122
Films, 78
Flyers, 144
Focus groups, 10-11
Folkman, S., 206, 207, 210
Formative evaluation, 21
Fries, J. F., 197
Fry formula, 123
Fund-raising, 148-149

Global helplessness, 213
Glucose monitoring, 84, 120
Groups, 8, 78-81, 88-90
    participation encouragement,
        174-176

Hard to help patients, 173-182
    antagonistic, 178
    attention seekers, 180-181
    special problems, 181
    strong, silent types, 174-176
    talkers, 176-178
    "Yes, buts," 179, 219
Health Assessment Questionnaire,
    49-57
Health belief model, 207, 215,
    222-224. *See also* Patient beliefs
Health professionals, 87-88
    marketing educational programs
        to, 132-136
Helplessness perceptions, 212-216
Hot-cold theory of disease, 163
Houland, C. I., 199, 222
Humor, 204
Hypertension, self-monitoring, 84

Implementation. *See* Planning and
    implementation
Instructor/facilitator, 85, 92
Instruments, 32. *See also* Scales
Interested-party analysis, 2-4, 132
Internality, 213
Interviews, needs assessment, 11-12

Joint Commission on Accreditation
    of Healthcare Organizations
    (JCAHO), 227-234

Keefe, F. J., 210

Language issues, 119, 155
    JCAHO guidelines, 230
    readability formulas, 123
    translation, 165, 166-170
Lazarus, R. S., 206, 207, 210
Learned helplessness, 200, 212-215
Lectures, 6-8
Life span, 197
Literacy, 159
Local adaptations, 133
Local media, 77
Locus-of-control theory, 200

Maier, S., 212
Marketing and promotion, 131-150
    community resources, 146-149
    hard to reach groups, 145-146
    to health professionals, 132-136
    to public, 136-146
    using media, 141, 144-145, 147
Mass media, 141, 144-145
Mastery, 201
Materials, 117-129
    field testing, 122

patient comprehension of, 119,
121-128
patient needs and, 118-121
Suitability Assessment, 125-128
translating, 165, 166-170
value of, 118
Media, 76-78, 147, 203-204
program marketing and, 141,
144-145
See also Materials
Medline, 32
Memory aids, 190-191
Mental health problems, 181
Models for behavior, 202-204
Models of patient education,
195-196
PRECEDE, 217-222
Morbidity, compression of, 197
Music, 165

Naming educational programs,
138, 166
Needs assessment, 1-17
balanced incomplete block
design, 12-16
checklist, 4-5
data analysis tool, 17
educational materials and,
118-119
focus groups, 10-11
interested-party analysis, 2-4
JCAHO regulations, 230
matrix, 8-9
salient beliefs assessment, 5-8
structured interviews, 11-12
Newsletters, 134, 144
NIH syndrome, 133

Objective(s), 71-75
Objective data, 23-24

Open-ended questions, 22-23, 82,
97, 174-175
Opening session, 91-92
Outcome evaluation, 21
Outcome objectives, 72
Outreach, 145-146. *See also*
Marketing and promotion
Ownership of educational
programs, 132, 133

Pain management, 187
Pain Visual Analogue Scale, 47
Participation-encouraging
techniques, 174-176
Patient, "hard to help" types. *See*
Hard to help patients
Patient beliefs, 187, 205
changing, 217-218
health belief model, 207, 215,
222-224
health misconceptions or myths,
161-162
predisposing factors, 217
salient beliefs, 5-8, 199
self-efficacy, 199-206
Patient education:
arthritis self-help course
protocol, 100-115
community resources, 146-149
definition and purpose of, xiii-xiv
JCAHO guidelines, 227-234
rationale, 195, 197
time and place, 140-141
Patient education models, 195-196
health beliefs, 215, 222-224
PRECEDE, 217-222
Patient education program
evaluation. *See* Evaluation
Patient education skills, 86-87
Patient education theories. *See*
Theories

Patient needs. *See* Needs assessment
Patient satisfaction, 62-65
Perceived threat, 222
Persuasion, 205
Planned educational activities, xiv-xv
Planning and implementation, 67
   content and skills, 86-87
   documentation, 95-96
   methods, 75-85
   objectives, 71-75
   priority setting, 68-70
   protocol preparation guidelines,
      90-95
   refining content, 71
Positive reappraisal, 210
Power struggles, 178
Prayer, 211
Predisposing factors, 217-219
Press releases, 141-143
Priority setting, 68-70, 120
Problem solving, 186, 210, 220
Process evaluation, 21
Process objectives, 72
Program content, 86-87
   refining, 71
Program evaluation. *See* Evaluation
Program implementation. *See*
      Planning and implementation
Program planning. *See* Planning
      and implementation
Promotion. *See* Marketing and
      promotion
Psychology Abstracts, 32
Publicity, 141, 144-145. *See also*
      Marketing and promotion
Public service announcements, 76,
      141

Qualitative evaluation methods,
      22-23, 26, 27-29
Quality of Life Visual Analogue
      Scale, 47-48

Quantitative evaluation methods,
      22, 26, 29-30
Question(s) and questioning,
      22-23, 29, 81-82, 97-99,
      174-175
   in evaluation scales, 32-35
Questionnaire design, 35-42

Radio, 144
Randomized comparison group,
      43-44
Range-of-motion exercises, 186-187
Rationale for patient education,
      195, 197
Reach for Recovery, 202
Readability formula, 122-125
Recruitment. *See* Marketing and
      promotion
Regulatory issues, JCAHO
      guidelines, 227-234
Rehearsal, 81
Reimbursement, 138-140
Reinforcement, 94-95, 175, 220-221
Reliability, 24
Resources, 91, 219, 220
Response burden, 30
Responsibility, 210
Ritual, 93
Role models, 166, 202-203
Role playing, 80
Rosenstiel, A. R., 210

Salient beliefs, 5-8, 199. *See also*
      Patient beliefs
Satisfaction Survey, 62-65
Scales, 32-34, 46-65
   consumer satisfaction, 62-65
   depression, 58-60
   health assessment, 49-57
   medication taking, 61
   visual analogue, 47-48

Self-control, 209
Self-efficacy, 31-32, 100, 192-193,
    199-206
Self-help course protocol, 100-115
Self-management, xiv, 94
Self-monitoring, 82-85, 87-88
Self-report, 23
Self-Reported Medication Taking
    Scale, 61
Self-talk, 211
Seligman, M., 212
Service clubs, 147
Sesame Street approach, 93
Settings, 140-141, 146-147
Situational appraisal, 207
Skills mastery, 201-202, 220
Sleepers, 176
Sliding scales, 139
Social support, 191, 209, 220
Software, 17
Spanish language speakers, 119,
    121, 155
Specific helplessness, 213
Stable attributions, 213
Statistics, 38
Stress and coping, 206-212
Strong, silent types, 174-176
Structured/semistructured
    interviews, 11-12
Study design, 42-44
Subjective data, 23-24
Suitability Assessment of Materials,
    125-128
Summative evaluation, 21
Support groups, 202
Support network, 191, 209, 220

Symptom reinterpretation, 204-205

Talkers, 176-178
Target behaviors, 68-70
Teaching priorities, 68-70
Teaching skills, 86-87
Theories, 195-196, 198-199
    learned helplessness, 200,
        212-215
    self-efficacy, 199-206
    stress and coping, 206-212
Time of program sessions, 140
Time utilization, 87
Trait-state distinction, 214
Translation, 165, 166-170

Understandability. See
    Comprehensibility
Unstable attributions, 214

Validity, 24
Videotapes, 78
Visual analogue scales, 47-48

Walking programs, 148
Weight monitoring, 85
Whiners, 180
Word of mouth, 145

"Yes, but," types of patients, 179,
    219

About the Author

Kate Lorig, Dr.P.H., RN, is an Associate Professor (Research) at Stanford University School of Medicine and is also Director of the Stanford Patient Education Research Center. She has spent the past 17 years developing and evaluating community-based patient education programs for people with chronic diseases.

She has also acted as a consultant for major HMOs, hospitals, and voluntary health agencies. Her programs have been adapted by other countries, including Canada, Australia, New Zealand, Great Britain, and South Africa.

About the
Contributing Coauthors

Cecilia Doak, M.P.H., is, with Leonard Doak, a founder of Patient Learning Associates, Inc., and is one of the foremost experts in the United States on the preparation of health education materials.

Leonard Doak, B.S., P.E., is, with Cecilia Doak, a founder of Patient Learning Associates, Inc., and is one of the foremost experts in the United States on the preparation of health education materials.

Jean Goeppinger, RN, Ph.D., is Chair of Community Health Nursing at the University of North Carolina at Chapel Hill. She received her Ph.D. in sociology from the University of Indiana.

Virginia M. González, M.P.H., is a Research Assistant at the Stanford Patient Education Research Center. She received her M.P.H. from the University of California at Berkeley.

Mary M. Hobbs, M.P.H., is the Director of Health Education for Kaiser Permanente Medical Group in Redwood City, California. She received her M.P.H. in health education from San Jose State University.